The Reflexology Planner

For a busy Reflexologist

Half Year Planner

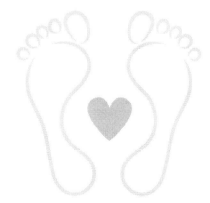

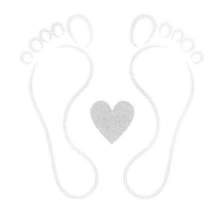

First Edition August 2021
www.katiepage.co.uk

Personal Information

This Book Belongs to: Samantha Robinson
Samantha Claire Therapies.

Telephone Number: 07786 570 600

Website:

Email Address: Samctherapies @ gmail. com.

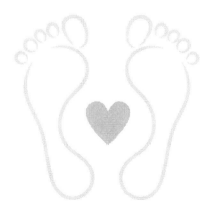

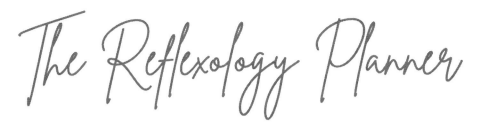

The Reflexology Planner

I am delighted that you are using The Reflexology Planner.

The Reflexology Planner is here to help you:

- Plan your weekly content
- Keep track of your Reflexology Business and Selfcare
- See your Business Development in one place
- To get more Visible
- To ensure you practice what you preach as a Reflexologist

Inside you will find:

- Weekly, Monthly and Quarterly checks
- Plan your wins
- Achieve your Intentions
- Remember your Self Care and its importance
- Celebrate your Success
- Footstep Challenge

Fill in the planner with all your Intentions, Aspirations and Actuals

Selfcare is important to your business. Included are:

- Reminders
- Gratitude
- Plan your celebrations
- Affirmations
- Journaling

Time to create a firmer footing in your business

Weekly Checks

Write your own Positive Affirmation to keep YOU focused, some are there for you
Write down 5 actions you must achieve this week
Social Media Follower tally
Numbers and Financials Goals
Socials Media Theme, Subjects & Hashtags
Where have you posted your Social Media Content?
What is your one Self Care checks and non negotiable
What were your Wins Of The Week?
Have you Journaled your week?
Habit Tracker
Celebrate your weekly wins

Monthly Checks

Monthly Checklist
Monthly Counts :
- Has your social media growth
- Has your turnover per client increased?
- Is your monthly client list growing?
Plan your Monthly Win
Footstep Challenge
Create your own positive affirmation for the month.

Quarterly Checks

Reflection on what went well
What could you have done differently
Quarterly Social Media Growth
Quarterly Client and Finance Checker
To Do Lists for the next Quarter

Date :

Months started:

Social Media Starting Point

Fill this out at the end of every Friday:

	Facebook Page A	Facebook Group B	Instagram C	Total A+B+C	Growth on previous month
Week 1					0
Week 2					
Week 3					
Week 4					
Week 5					
Week 6					
Week 7					
Week 8					
Week 9					
Week 10					
Week 11					
Week 12					
TOTALS					

Date :

Months started:

Client Growth Starting Point

Fill this out at the end of every Friday:

	No of Clients A	No of New Clients B	WeeklyTurnover C	Turnover per client C/A
Week 1				
Week 2				
Week 3				
Week 4				
Week 5				
Week 6				
Week 7				
Week 8				
Week 9				
Week 10				
Week 11				
Week 12				
TOTALS				

Date:

Plot, by colouring in, your level of business and wellbeing in each area on a scale of 1 - 10.
1 being the first foot and not so good and 10 being the last foot and top totch:

Personal Development - Training, Reading & Learning

Exercise and Diet - Maybe Yoga, Pilates, Walking or Running and the fuel you supply to your body to enable you to be effective

Sleep - Napping or Sleeping

Finances, ie Accounts, Paying yourself etc

Social inc Networking & Business Interaction

Downtime - Time you spend with Family and Friends

Emotional Well Being

Fun & Celebrating

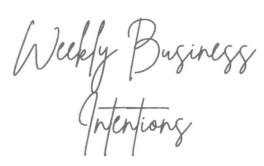

Start on a Monday

Month:

Week:

Weekly Business Intentions

I must achieve this week:

1. ....

2. ....

3. ....

4. ....

5. ....

How many followers do you have:

Facebook Page: ....

Facebook Group: ....

Instagram: ....

LinkedIn: ....

Affirmation:

Today starts with me I will have an amazing week

Numbers:

What is my Financial Goal for the week?

How many clients would you like to see?   How many new clients would you like to see?

How will you achieve the numbers above:

....

....

....

Theme for the Week:

What subjects can you break your theme into subjects:

Monday:

Tuesday:

Wednesday:

Thursday:

Friday:

Weekend:

Social Media Locations:

Colour in the hearts when the content is posted or scheduled

	M	T	W	T	F	S	S
Facebook Page	♡	♡	♡	♡	♡	♡	♡
Facebook Group	♡	♡	♡	♡	♡	♡	♡
Facebook Live	♡	♡	♡	♡	♡	♡	♡
Instagram	♡	♡	♡	♡	♡	♡	♡
Instagram Stories	♡	♡	♡	♡	♡	♡	♡
LinkedIn	♡	♡	♡	♡	♡	♡	♡
Twitter	♡	♡	♡	♡	♡	♡	♡
Google	♡	♡	♡	♡	♡	♡	♡

Theme for the week Hashtags:

Month:

Week:

Weekly Business Checks and Selfcare

Selfcare Checks:

Colour in the hearts when you have achieved each self care step.

Colour in one for once and both for more than once.

Have you:

Exercised	♡	♡
Journaled	♡	♡
Affirmed your Affirmation	♡	♡
5 minutes Silence	♡	♡
Visualised where you want to be by the end of the week	♡	♡
Written down 5 things a day you are grateful for	♡	♡
Meditation	♡	♡
Set my Intentions for the week	♡	♡
Read a book	♡	♡

I am grateful for:

1.

2.

3.

4.

5.

What will you do to celebrate the week?

What is your ONE selfcare non negotiable this week?

What was your unexpected WIN of the week?

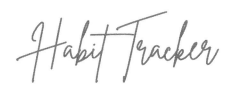

Habit Tracker

Habit trackers are exactly what they say they are. Map out your footsteps to keeping your new habits on track:

Where are you now?

Colour in how well you are doing today

This wheel is the start of your footsteps to creating some great habits to help you keep your business on sturdy footings.

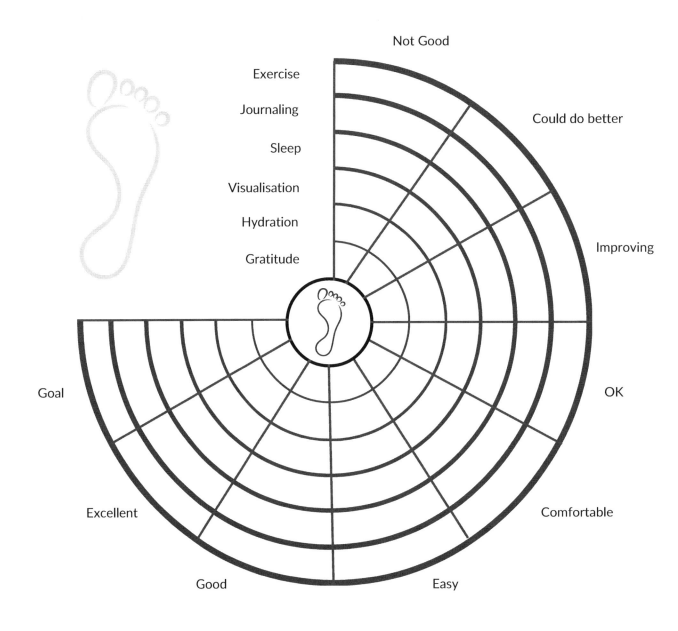

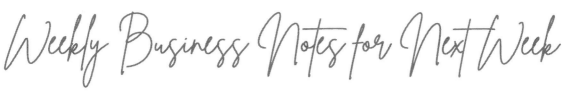

Weekly Business Notes for Next Week

_____

_____

_____

_____

_____

_____

_____

_____

_____

_____

_____

_____

_____

_____

_____

_____

Month:

Week:

Weekly Business Intentions

I must achieve this week:

1. ....

2. ....

3. ....

4. ....

5. ....

How many followers do you have:

Facebook Page: ....

Facebook Group: ....

Instagram: ....

LinkedIn: ....

Affirmation:

I have the power to change my thoughts

Numbers:

What is my Financial Goal for the week?

How many clients would you like to see?   How many new clients would you like to see?

How will you achieve the numbers above:

....

....

....

Theme for the Week:

Weekly Social Media Planning

What subjects can you break your theme into subjects:

Monday:

Tuesday:

Wednesday:

Thursday:

Friday:

Weekend:

Social Media Locations:

Colour in the hearts when the content is posted or scheduled

	M	T	W	T	F	S	S
Facebook Page	♡	♡	♡	♡	♡	♡	♡
Facebook Group	♡	♡	♡	♡	♡	♡	♡
Facebook Live	♡	♡	♡	♡	♡	♡	♡
Instagram	♡	♡	♡	♡	♡	♡	♡
Instagram Stories	♡	♡	♡	♡	♡	♡	♡
LinkedIn	♡	♡	♡	♡	♡	♡	♡
Twitter	♡	♡	♡	♡	♡	♡	♡
Google	♡	♡	♡	♡	♡	♡	♡

Theme for the week Hashtags:

Month:

Week:

Weekly Business Checks and Selfcare

Selfcare Checks:

Colour in the hearts when you have achieved each self care step.

Colour in one for once and both for more than once.

Have you:

Exercised ♡ ♡

Journaled ♡ ♡

Affirmed your Affirmation ♡ ♡

5 minutes Silence ♡ ♡

Visualised where you want to be by the end of the week ♡ ♡

Written down 5 things a day you are grateful for ♡ ♡

Meditation ♡ ♡

Set my Intentions for the week ♡ ♡

Read a book ♡ ♡

I am grateful for:

1.

2.

3.

4.

5.

What will you do to celebrate the week?

What is your ONE selfcare non negotiable this week?

What was your unexpected WIN of the week?

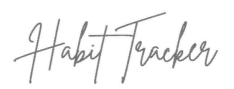

Habit Tracker

Habit trackers are exactly what they say they are. Map out your footsteps to keeping your new habits on track:

Where are you now?

Colour in how well you are doing today

This wheel is the start of your footsteps to creating some great habits to help you keep your business on sturdy footings.

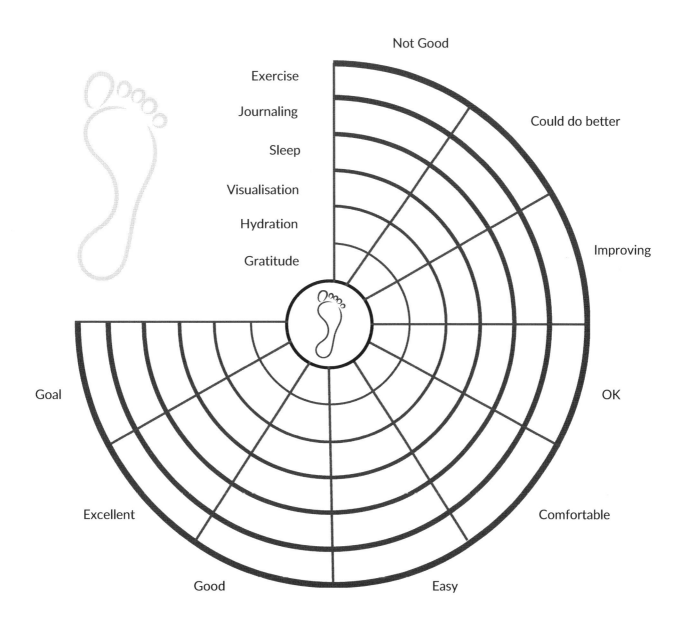

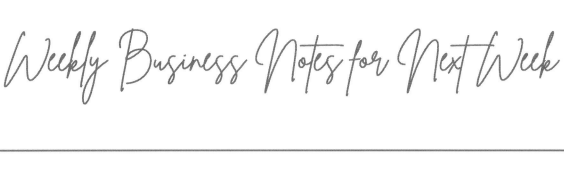

Weekly Business Notes for Next Week

Month:

Week:

Weekly Business Intentions

I must achieve this week:

1. ....

2. ....

3. ....

4. ....

5. ....

How many followers do you have:

Facebook Page: ....

Facebook Group: ....

Instagram: ....

LinkedIn: ....

Affirmation:

This week will be the best I can make it

Numbers:

What is my Financial Goal for the week?

How many clients would you like to see?   How many new clients would you like to see?

How will you achieve the numbers above:

....

....

....

Theme for the Week:

*Weekly Social
Media Planning*

What subjects can you break your theme into subjects:

Monday:

Tuesday:

Wednesday:

Thursday:

Friday:

Weekend:

Social Media Locations:

Colour in the hearts when the content is posted or scheduled

	M	T	W	T	F	S	S
Facebook Page	♡	♡	♡	♡	♡	♡	♡
Facebook Group	♡	♡	♡	♡	♡	♡	♡
Facebook Live	♡	♡	♡	♡	♡	♡	♡
Instagram	♡	♡	♡	♡	♡	♡	♡
Instagram Stories	♡	♡	♡	♡	♡	♡	♡
LinkedIn	♡	♡	♡	♡	♡	♡	♡
Twitter	♡	♡	♡	♡	♡	♡	♡
Google	♡	♡	♡	♡	♡	♡	♡

Theme for the week Hashtags:

Month:

Week:

Weekly Business Checks and Selfcare

Selfcare Checks:

Colour in the hearts when you have achieved each self care step.

Colour in one for once and both for more than once.

Have you:

Exercised ♡ ♡

Journaled ♡ ♡

Affirmed your Affirmation ♡ ♡

5 minutes Silence ♡ ♡

Visualised where you want to be by the end of the week ♡ ♡

Written down 5 things a day you are grateful for ♡ ♡

Meditation ♡ ♡

Set my Intentions for the week ♡ ♡

Read a book ♡ ♡

I am grateful for:

1.

2.

3.

4.

5.

What will you do to celebrate the week?

What is your ONE selfcare non negotiable this week?

What was your unexpected WIN of the week?

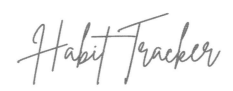

Habit Tracker

Habit trackers are exactly what they say they are. Map out your footsteps to keeping your new habits on track:

Where are you now?

Colour in how well you are doing today

This wheel is the start of your footsteps to creating some great habits to help you keep your business on sturdy footings.

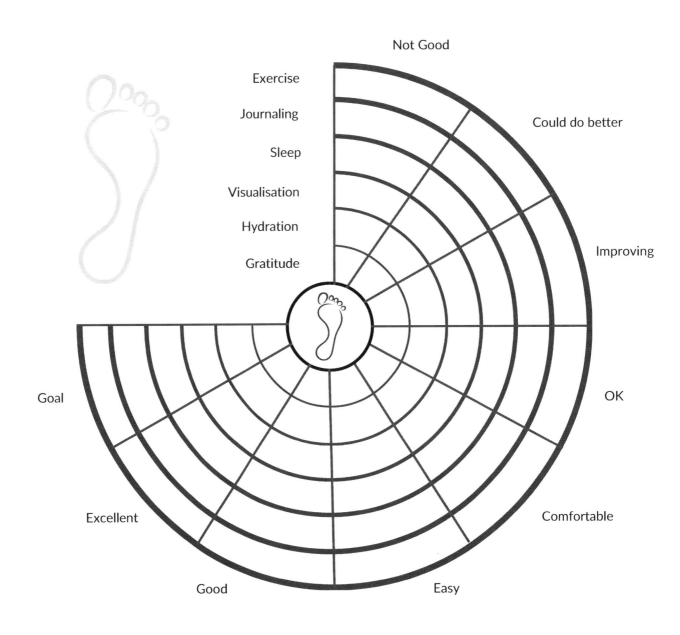

Weekly Business Notes for Next Week

Month:

Week:

I must achieve this week:

1. ....

2. ....

3. ....

4. ....

5. ....

How many followers do you have:

Facebook Page: ....

Facebook Group: ....

Instagram: ....

LinkedIn: ....

Affirmation:

My self belief has no boundaries

Numbers:

What is my Financial Goal for the week?

How many clients would you like to see?   How many new clients would you like to see?

How will you achieve the numbers above:

....

....

....

Theme for the Week:

Weekly Social Media Planning

What subjects can you break your theme into subjects:

Monday:

Tuesday:

Wednesday:

Thursday:

Friday:

Weekend:

Social Media Locations:

Colour in the hearts when the content is posted or scheduled

	M	T	W	T	F	S	S
Facebook Page	♡	♡	♡	♡	♡	♡	♡
Facebook Group	♡	♡	♡	♡	♡	♡	♡
Facebook Live	♡	♡	♡	♡	♡	♡	♡
Instagram	♡	♡	♡	♡	♡	♡	♡
Instagram Stories	♡	♡	♡	♡	♡	♡	♡
LinkedIn	♡	♡	♡	♡	♡	♡	♡
Twitter	♡	♡	♡	♡	♡	♡	♡
Google	♡	♡	♡	♡	♡	♡	♡

Theme for the week Hashtags:

Month:

Week:

Selfcare Checks:

Colour in the hearts when you have achieved each self care step.

Colour in one for once and both for more than once.

Have you:

Exercised ♡ ♡

Journaled ♡ ♡

Affirmed your Affirmation ♡ ♡

5 minutes Silence ♡ ♡

Visualised where you want to be by the end of the week ♡ ♡

Written down 5 things a day you are grateful for ♡ ♡

Meditation ♡ ♡

Set my Intentions for the week ♡ ♡

Read a book ♡ ♡

I am grateful for:

1.

2.

3.

4.

5.

What will you do to celebrate the week?

What is your ONE selfcare non negotiable this week?

What was your unexpected WIN of the week?

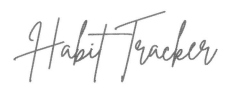

Habit Tracker

Habit trackers are exactly what they say they are. Map out your footsteps to keeping your new habits on track:

Where are you now?

Colour in how well you are doing today

This wheel is the start of your footsteps to creating some great habits to help you keep your business on sturdy footings.

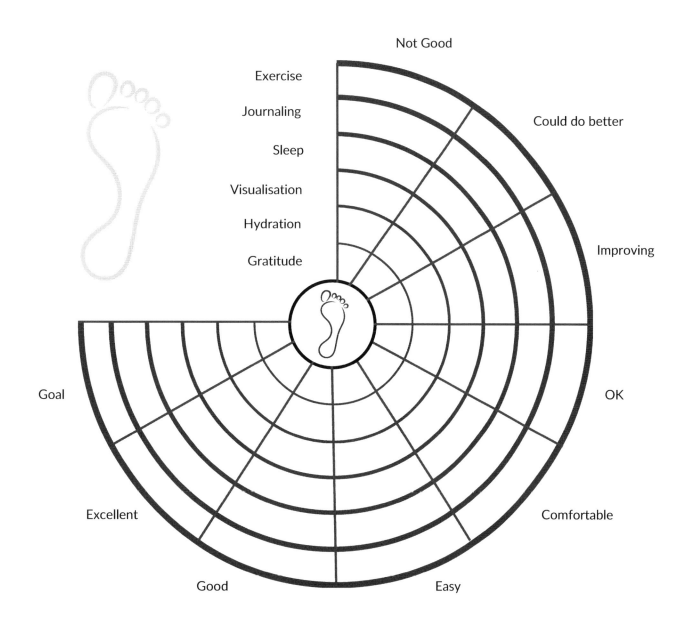

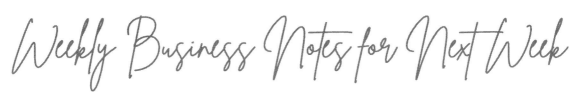

Weekly Business Notes for Next Week

Month:

Week:

Weekly Business Intentions

I must achieve this week:

1. ....

2. ....

3. ....

4. ....

5. ....

How many followers do you have:

Facebook Page: ....

Facebook Group: ....

Instagram: ....

LinkedIn: ....

Affirmation:

I will make my dreams a reality

Numbers:

What is my Financial Goal for the week?

How many clients would you like to see?   How many new clients would you like to see?

How will you achieve the numbers above:

....

....

....

Theme for the Week:

What subjects can you break your theme into subjects:

Monday:

Tuesday:

Wednesday:

Thursday:

Friday:

Weekend:

Social Media Locations:

Colour in the hearts when the content is posted or scheduled

	M	T	W	T	F	S	S
Facebook Page	♡	♡	♡	♡	♡	♡	♡
Facebook Group	♡	♡	♡	♡	♡	♡	♡
Facebook Live	♡	♡	♡	♡	♡	♡	♡
Instagram	♡	♡	♡	♡	♡	♡	♡
Instagram Stories	♡	♡	♡	♡	♡	♡	♡
LinkedIn	♡	♡	♡	♡	♡	♡	♡
Twitter	♡	♡	♡	♡	♡	♡	♡
Google	♡	♡	♡	♡	♡	♡	♡

Theme for the week Hashtags:

Month:

Week:

Selfcare Checks:

Colour in the hearts when you have achieved each self care step.

Colour in one for once and both for more than once.

Have you:

Exercised ♡ ♡

Journaled ♡ ♡

Affirmed your Affirmation ♡ ♡

5 minutes Silence ♡ ♡

Visualised where you want to be by the end of the week ♡ ♡

Written down 5 things a day you are grateful for ♡ ♡

Meditation ♡ ♡

Set my Intentions for the week ♡ ♡

Read a book ♡ ♡

I am grateful for:

1.

2.

3.

4.

5.

What will you do to celebrate the week?

What is your ONE selfcare non negotiable this week?

What was your unexpected WIN of the week?

Habit Tracker

Habit trackers are exactly what they say they are. Map out your footsteps to keeping your new habits on track:

Where are you now?

Colour in how well you are doing today

This wheel is the start of your footsteps to creating some great habits to help you keep your business on sturdy footings.

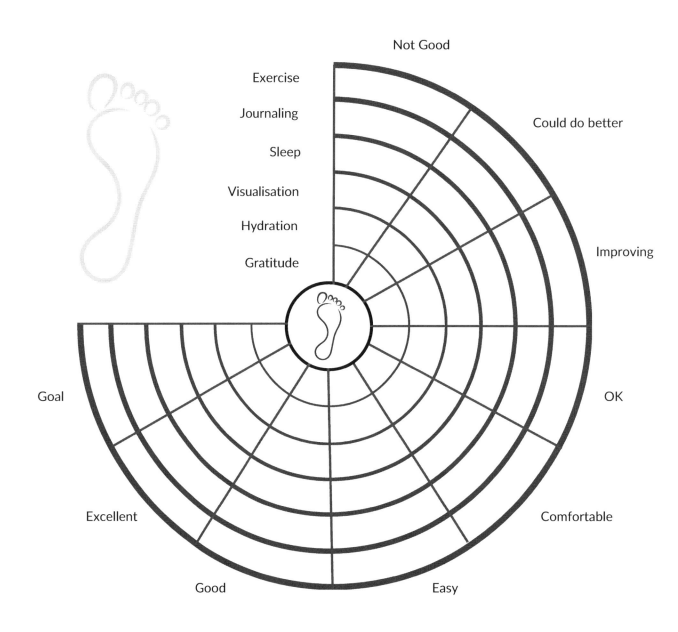

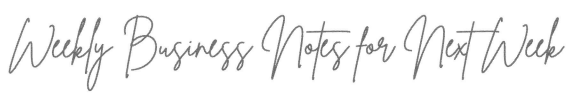

Weekly Business Notes for Next Week

Month:

Week:

Monthly Business Checks Up

Monthly Checks:

Colour in the hearts when you have achieved each self care step.

Have you:

1. Updated your website ♡
2. Written a blog ♡
3. Read an inspirational book ♡
4. Gone "Live" on Facebook ♡
5. Done a "Reel" on Instagram ♡
6. Preschedule your posts for next month ♡
7. Planned your socials for next month ♡
8. Exercised each day/week ♡
9. Increased your Tax Savings Bank Account ♡
10. Booked a month end Celebration ♡
11. Paid all your invoices ♡
12. Are your accounts up to date ♡
13. Did your social media grow ♡
14. Did your client list grow ♡
15. Pay yourself ♡
16. Met up with a business colleague ♡
17. Attended a networking event ♡
18. Organised a treat for YOU ♡
19. Achieved your financial goals ♡
20. Increased your costs per client ♡

This month I am grateful for:

1.

2.

3.

4.

5.

What was your unexpected WIN of the month?

What will you do to celebrate next month?

Journal your Thoughts of the Month:

Month:

Prompts:

What was good,
What could I have improved on,
What have I enjoyed,
What questions do I need to ask,
Who can I connect with.

Journal your Thoughts of the Month:

My To Do List:

_____
_____
_____
_____
_____
_____
_____
_____
_____
_____
_____
_____
_____

My Personal Affirmation for the month:

Date:

Plot, by colouring in, your level of business and wellbeing in each area on a scale of 1 - 10.
1 being the first foot and not so good and 10 being the last foot and top totch:

Personal Development - Training, Reading &
Learning

Exercise and Diet - Maybe Yoga, Pilates, Walking
or Running and the fuel you supply to your body to
enable you to be effective

Sleep - Napping or Sleeping

Finances, ie Accounts, Paying yourself etc

Social inc Networking & Business Interaction

Downtime - Time you spend with Family and Friends

Emotional Well Being

Fun & Celebrating

Month:

Week:

Weekly Business Intentions

I must achieve this week:

1. ....
2. ....
3. ....
4. ....
5. ....

How many followers do you have:

Facebook Page: ....

Facebook Group: ....

Instagram: ....

LinkedIn: ....

Affirmation:

I can, I will and I am going to show you I can!.

Numbers:

What is my Financial Goal for the week?

How many clients would you like to see?   How many new clients would you like to see?

How will you achieve the numbers above:

....

....

....

Theme for the Week:

Weekly Social Media Planning

What subjects can you break your theme into subjects:

Monday:

Tuesday:

Wednesday:

Thursday:

Friday:

Weekend:

Social Media Locations:

Colour in the hearts when the content is posted or scheduled

	M	T	W	T	F	S	S
Facebook Page	♡	♡	♡	♡	♡	♡	♡
Facebook Group	♡	♡	♡	♡	♡	♡	♡
Facebook Live	♡	♡	♡	♡	♡	♡	♡
Instagram	♡	♡	♡	♡	♡	♡	♡
Instagram Stories	♡	♡	♡	♡	♡	♡	♡
LinkedIn	♡	♡	♡	♡	♡	♡	♡
Twitter	♡	♡	♡	♡	♡	♡	♡
Google	♡	♡	♡	♡	♡	♡	♡

Theme for the week Hashtags:

Month:

Week:

Selfcare Checks:

Colour in the hearts when you have achieved each self care step.

Colour in one for once and both for more than once.

Have you:

Exercised ♡ ♡

Journaled ♡ ♡

Affirmed your Affirmation ♡ ♡

5 minutes Silence ♡ ♡

Visualised where you want to be by the end of the week ♡ ♡

Written down 5 things a day you are grateful for ♡ ♡

Meditation ♡ ♡

Set my Intentions for the week ♡ ♡

Read a book ♡ ♡

I am grateful for:

1.

2.

3.

4.

5.

What will you do to celebrate the week?

What is your ONE selfcare non negotiable this week?

What was your unexpected WIN of the week?

Habit Tracker
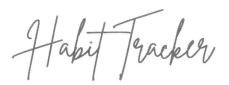

Habit trackers are exactly what they say they are. Map out your footsteps to keeping your new habits on track:

Where are you now?

Colour in how well you are doing today

This wheel is the start of your footsteps to creating some great habits to help you keep your business on sturdy footings.

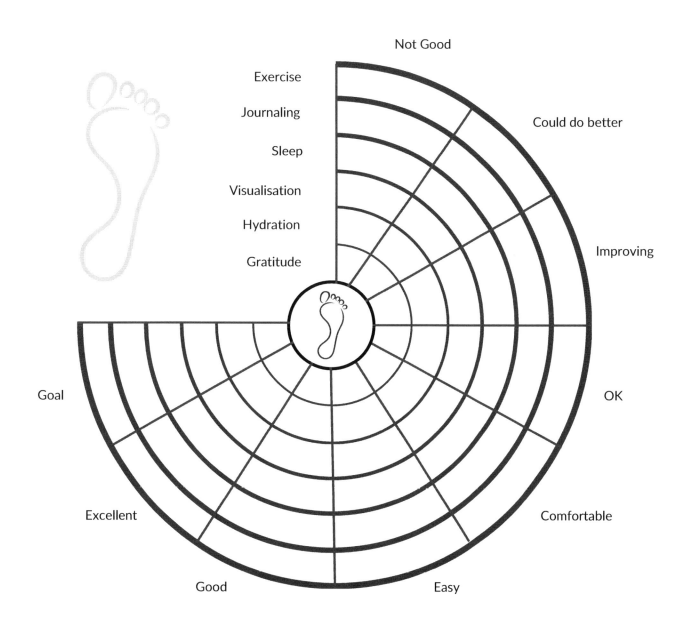

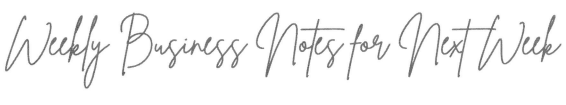

Weekly Business Notes for Next Week

Month:

Week:

Weekly Business Intentions

I must achieve this week:

1. ....

2. ....

3. ....

4. ....

5. ....

How many followers do you have:

Facebook Page: ....

Facebook Group: ....

Instagram: ....

LinkedIn: ....

Affirmation:

I am overcoming my fears to realise my dreams.

Numbers:

What is my Financial Goal for the week?

How many clients would you like to see?   How many new clients would you like to see?

How will you achieve the numbers above:

....

....

....

Theme for the Week:

Weekly Social Media Planning

What subjects can you break your theme into subjects:

Monday:

Tuesday:

Wednesday:

Thursday:

Friday:

Weekend:

Social Media Locations:

Colour in the hearts when the content is posted or scheduled

	M	T	W	T	F	S	S
Facebook Page	♡	♡	♡	♡	♡	♡	♡
Facebook Group	♡	♡	♡	♡	♡	♡	♡
Facebook Live	♡	♡	♡	♡	♡	♡	♡
Instagram	♡	♡	♡	♡	♡	♡	♡
Instagram Stories	♡	♡	♡	♡	♡	♡	♡
LinkedIn	♡	♡	♡	♡	♡	♡	♡
Twitter	♡	♡	♡	♡	♡	♡	♡
Google	♡	♡	♡	♡	♡	♡	♡

Theme for the week Hashtags:

Month:

Week:

Selfcare Checks:

Colour in the hearts when you have achieved each self care step.

Colour in one for once and both for more than once.

Have you:

Exercised ♡ ♡

Journaled ♡ ♡

Affirmed your Affirmation ♡ ♡

5 minutes Silence ♡ ♡

Visualised where you want to be by the end of the week ♡ ♡

Written down 5 things a day you are grateful for ♡ ♡

Meditation ♡ ♡

Set my Intentions for the week ♡ ♡

Read a book ♡ ♡

I am grateful for:

1.

2.

3.

4.

5.

What will you do to celebrate the week?

What is your ONE selfcare non negotiable this week?

What was your unexpected WIN of the week?

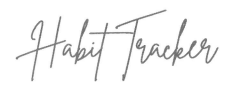

Habit Tracker

Habit trackers are exactly what they say they are. Map out your footsteps to keeping your new habits on track:

Where are you now?

Colour in how well you are doing today

This wheel is the start of your footsteps to creating some great habits to help you keep your business on sturdy footings.

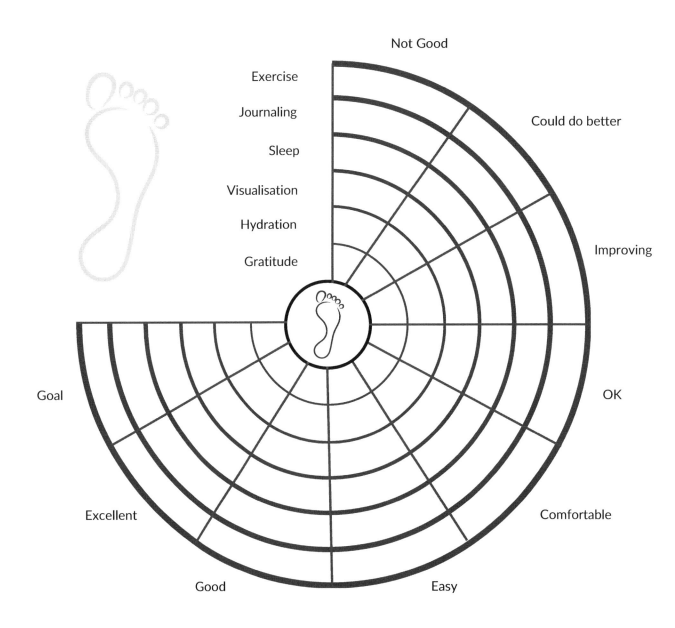

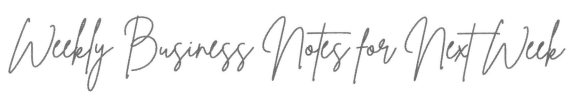

Weekly Business Notes for Next Week

Month:

Week:

I must achieve this week:

1. ....

2. ....

3. ....

4. ....

5. ....

How many followers do you have:

Facebook Page: ....

Facebook Group: ....

Instagram: ....

LinkedIn: ....

Affirmation:

I am a fabulous at my job

Numbers:

What is my Financial Goal for the week?

How many clients would you like to see?   How many new clients would you like to see?

How will you achieve the numbers above:

....

....

....

Theme for the Week:

Weekly Social Media Planning

What subjects can you break your theme into subjects:

Monday:

Tuesday:

Wednesday:

Thursday:

Friday:

Weekend:

Social Media Locations:

Colour in the hearts when the content is posted or scheduled

	M	T	W	T	F	S	S
Facebook Page	♡	♡	♡	♡	♡	♡	♡
Facebook Group	♡	♡	♡	♡	♡	♡	♡
Facebook Live	♡	♡	♡	♡	♡	♡	♡
Instagram	♡	♡	♡	♡	♡	♡	♡
Instagram Stories	♡	♡	♡	♡	♡	♡	♡
LinkedIn	♡	♡	♡	♡	♡	♡	♡
Twitter	♡	♡	♡	♡	♡	♡	♡
Google	♡	♡	♡	♡	♡	♡	♡

Theme for the week Hashtags:

Month:

Week:

Selfcare Checks:

Colour in the hearts when you have achieved each self care step.

Colour in one for once and both for more than once.

Have you:

Exercised ♡ ♡

Journaled ♡ ♡

Affirmed your Affirmation ♡ ♡

5 minutes Silence ♡ ♡

Visualised where you want to be by the end of the week ♡ ♡

Written down 5 things a day you are grateful for ♡ ♡

Meditation ♡ ♡

Set my Intentions for the week ♡ ♡

Read a book ♡ ♡

I am grateful for:

1.

2.

3.

4.

5.

What will you do to celebrate the week?

What is your ONE selfcare non negotiable this week?

What was your unexpected WIN of the week?

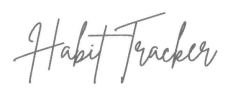

Habit Tracker

Habit trackers are exactly what they say they are. Map out your footsteps to keeping your new habits on track:

Where are you now?

Colour in how well you are doing today

This wheel is the start of your footsteps to creating some great habits to help you keep your business on sturdy footings.

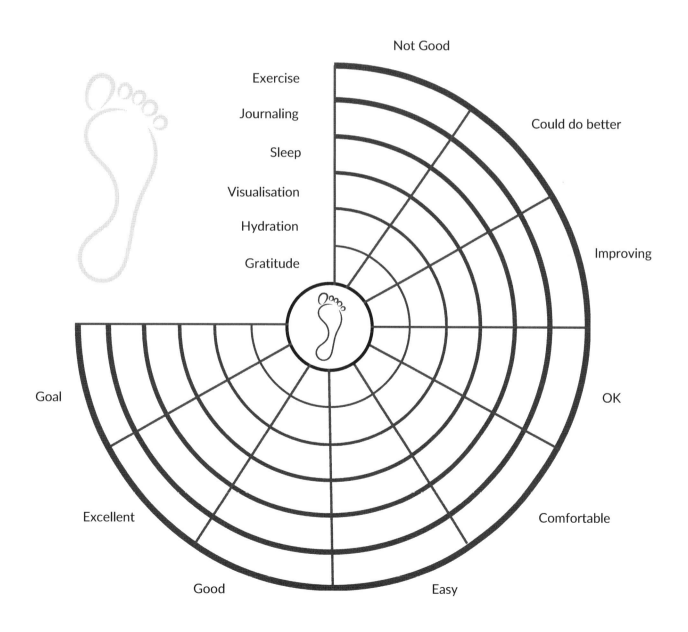

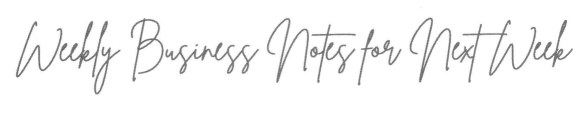

Weekly Business Notes for Next Week

Month:

Week:

Weekly Business Intentions

I must achieve this week:

1. ....

2. ....

3. ....

4. ....

5. ....

How many followers do you have:

Facebook Page: ....

Facebook Group: ....

Instagram: ....

LinkedIn: ....

Affirmation:

I will make the most of all new opportunities

Numbers:

What is my Financial Goal for the week?

How many clients would you like to see?   How many new clients would you like to see?

How will you achieve the numbers above:

....

....

....

Theme for the Week:

Weekly Social Media Planning

What subjects can you break your theme into subjects:

Monday:

Tuesday:

Wednesday:

Thursday:

Friday:

Weekend:

Social Media Locations:

Colour in the hearts when the content is posted or scheduled

	M	T	W	T	F	S	S
Facebook Page	♡	♡	♡	♡	♡	♡	♡
Facebook Group	♡	♡	♡	♡	♡	♡	♡
Facebook Live	♡	♡	♡	♡	♡	♡	♡
Instagram	♡	♡	♡	♡	♡	♡	♡
Instagram Stories	♡	♡	♡	♡	♡	♡	♡
LinkedIn	♡	♡	♡	♡	♡	♡	♡
Twitter	♡	♡	♡	♡	♡	♡	♡
Google	♡	♡	♡	♡	♡	♡	♡

Theme for the week Hashtags:

Month:

Week:

Selfcare Checks:

Colour in the hearts when you have achieved each self care step.

Colour in one for once and both for more than once.

Have you:

Exercised ♡ ♡

Journaled ♡ ♡

Affirmed your Affirmation ♡ ♡

5 minutes Silence ♡ ♡

Visualised where you want to be by the end of the week ♡ ♡

Written down 5 things a day you are grateful for ♡ ♡

Meditation ♡ ♡

Set my Intentions for the week ♡ ♡

Read a book ♡ ♡

I am grateful for:

1.

2.

3.

4.

5.

What will you do to celebrate the week?

What is your ONE selfcare non negotiable this week?

What was your unexpected WIN of the week?

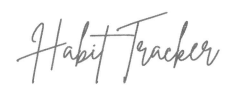

Habit Tracker

Habit trackers are exactly what they say they are. Map out your footsteps to keeping your new habits on track:

Where are you now?

Colour in how well you are doing today

This wheel is the start of your footsteps to creating some great habits to help you keep your business on sturdy footings.

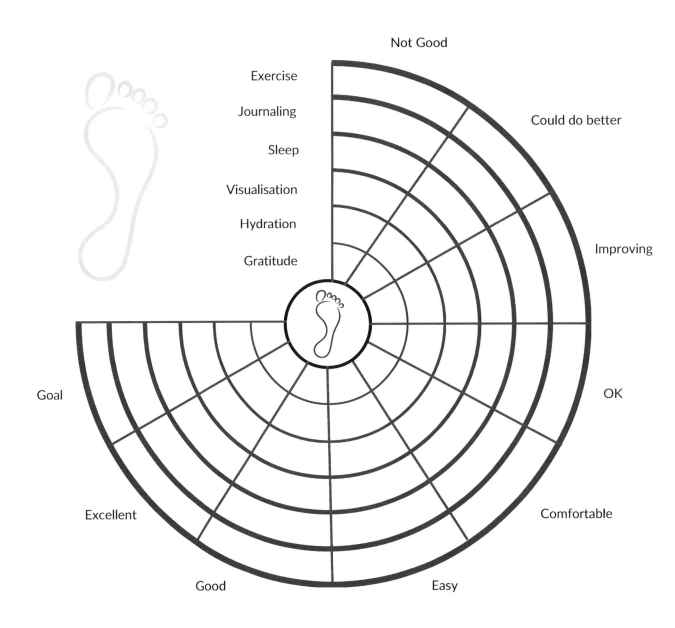

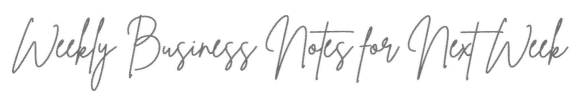

Weekly Business Notes for Next Week

Month:

Week:

Weekly Business Intentions

I must achieve this week:

1. ....

2. ....

3. ....

4. ....

5. ....

How many followers do you have:

Facebook Page: ....

Facebook Group: ....

Instagram: ....

LinkedIn: ....

Affirmation:

I feel safe in the rhythm and flow of my ever changing life

Numbers:

What is my Financial Goal for the week?

How many clients would you like to see?　　　　　How many new clients would you like to see?

How will you achieve the numbers above:

....

....

....

Theme for the Week:

What subjects can you break your theme into subjects:

Monday:

Tuesday:

Wednesday:

Thursday:

Friday:

Weekend:

Social Media Locations:

Colour in the hearts when the content is posted or scheduled

	M	T	W	T	F	S	S
Facebook Page	♡	♡	♡	♡	♡	♡	♡
Facebook Group	♡	♡	♡	♡	♡	♡	♡
Facebook Live	♡	♡	♡	♡	♡	♡	♡
Instagram	♡	♡	♡	♡	♡	♡	♡
Instagram Stories	♡	♡	♡	♡	♡	♡	♡
LinkedIn	♡	♡	♡	♡	♡	♡	♡
Twitter	♡	♡	♡	♡	♡	♡	♡
Google	♡	♡	♡	♡	♡	♡	♡

Theme for the week Hashtags:

Month:

Week:

Selfcare Checks:

Colour in the hearts when you have achieved each self care step.

Colour in one for once and both for more than once.

Have you:

Exercised ♡ ♡

Journaled ♡ ♡

Affirmed your Affirmation ♡ ♡

5 minutes Silence ♡ ♡

Visualised where you want to be by the end of the week ♡ ♡

Written down 5 things a day you are grateful for ♡ ♡

Meditation ♡ ♡

Set my Intentions for the week ♡ ♡

Read a book ♡ ♡

I am grateful for:

1.

2.

3.

4.

5.

What will you do to celebrate the week?

What is your ONE selfcare non negotiable this week?

What was your unexpected WIN of the week?

Habit Tracker

Habit trackers are exactly what they say they are. Map out your footsteps to keeping your new habits on track:

Where are you now?

Colour in how well you are doing today

This wheel is the start of your footsteps to creating some great habits to help you keep your business on sturdy footings.

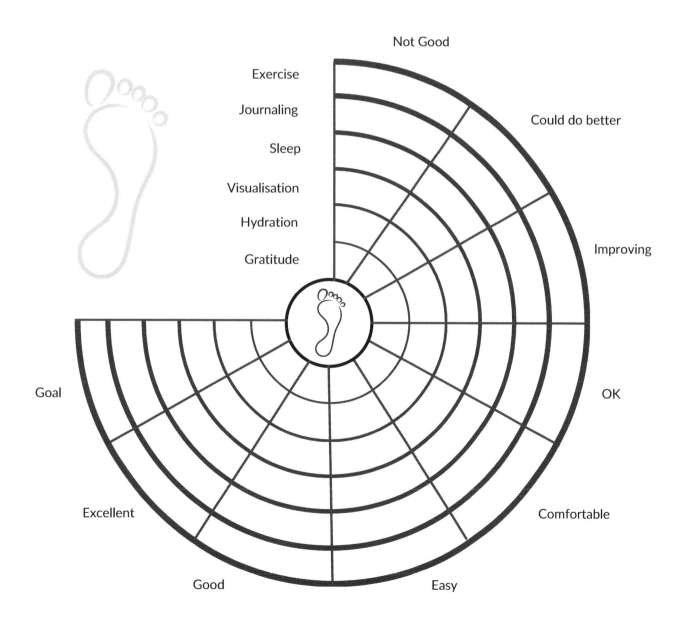

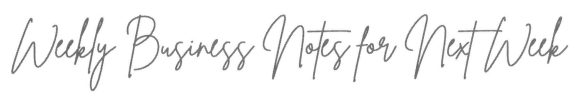

Weekly Business Notes for Next Week

Month:

Week:

Monthly Business Checks Up

Monthly Checks:

Colour in the hearts when you have achieved each self care step.

Have you:

1. Updated your website ♡
2. Written a blog ♡
3. Read an inspirational book ♡
4. Gone "Live" on Facebook ♡
5. Done a "Reel" on Instagram ♡
6. Preschedule your posts for next month ♡
7. Planned your socials for next month ♡
8. Exercised each day/week ♡
9. Increased your Tax Savings Bank Account ♡
10. Booked a month end Celebration ♡
11. Paid all your invoices ♡
12. Are your accounts up to date ♡
13. Did your social media grow ♡
14. Did your client list grow ♡
15. Pay yourself ♡
16. Met up with a business colleague ♡
17. Attended a networking event ♡
18. Organised a treat for YOU ♡
19. Achieved your financial goals ♡
20. Increased your costs per client ♡

This month I am grateful for:

1.

2.

3.

4.

5.

What was your unexpected WIN of the month?

What will you do to celebrate next month?

Journal your Thoughts of the Month:

_____

_____

_____

_____

Month:

Prompts:

What was good,
What could I have improved on,
What have I enjoyed,
What questions do I need to ask,
Who can I connect with.

_____

_____

_____

_____

_____

_____

_____

_____

_____

_____

_____

_____

_____

Journal your Thoughts of the Month:

My To Do List:

_____

_____

_____

_____

_____

_____

_____

_____

_____

My Personal Affirmation for the month:

Date:

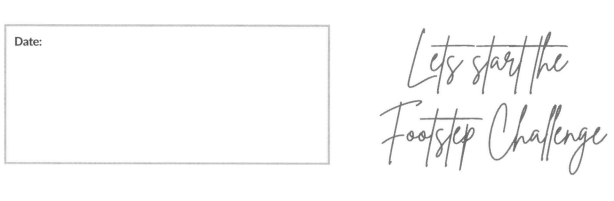

Plot, by colouring in, your level of business and wellbeing in each area on a scale of 1 - 10.
1 being the first foot and not so good and 10 being the last foot and top totch:

Personal Development - Training, Reading & Learning

Exercise and Diet - Maybe Yoga, Pilates, Walking or Running and the fuel you supply to your body to enable you to be effective

Sleep - Napping or Sleeping

Finances, ie Accounts, Paying yourself etc

Social inc Networking & Business Interaction

Downtime - Time you spend with Family and Friends

Emotional Well Being

Fun & Celebrating

Month:

Week:

I must achieve this week:

1. ....

2. ....

3. ....

4. ....

5. ....

How many followers do you have:

Facebook Page: ....

Facebook Group: ....

Instagram: ....

LinkedIn: ....

Affirmation:

I refuse to give up, I will be positive & happy all this week.

Numbers:

What is my Financial Goal for the week?

How many clients would you like to see?   How many new clients would you like to see?

How will you achieve the numbers above:

....

....

....

Theme for the Week:

Weekly Social Media Planning

What subjects can you break your theme into subjects:

Monday:

Tuesday:

Wednesday:

Thursday:

Friday:

Weekend:

Social Media Locations:

Colour in the hearts when the content is posted or scheduled

	M	T	W	T	F	S	S
Facebook Page	♡	♡	♡	♡	♡	♡	♡
Facebook Group	♡	♡	♡	♡	♡	♡	♡
Facebook Live	♡	♡	♡	♡	♡	♡	♡
Instagram	♡	♡	♡	♡	♡	♡	♡
Instagram Stories	♡	♡	♡	♡	♡	♡	♡
LinkedIn	♡	♡	♡	♡	♡	♡	♡
Twitter	♡	♡	♡	♡	♡	♡	♡
Google	♡	♡	♡	♡	♡	♡	♡

Theme for the week Hashtags:

Month:

Week:

Selfcare Checks:

Colour in the hearts when you have achieved each self care step.

Colour in one for once and both for more than once.

Have you:

Exercised

Journaled

Affirmed your Affirmation

5 minutes Silence

Visualised where you want to be by the end of the week

Written down 5 things a day you are grateful for

Meditation

Set my Intentions for the week

Read a book

I am grateful for:

1.

2.

3.

4.

5.

What will you do to celebrate the week?

What is your ONE selfcare non negotiable this week?

What was your unexpected WIN of the week?

Habit Tracker

Habit trackers are exactly what they say they are. Map out your footsteps to keeping your new habits on track:

Where are you now?

Colour in how well you are doing today

This wheel is the start of your footsteps to creating some great habits to help you keep your business on sturdy footings.

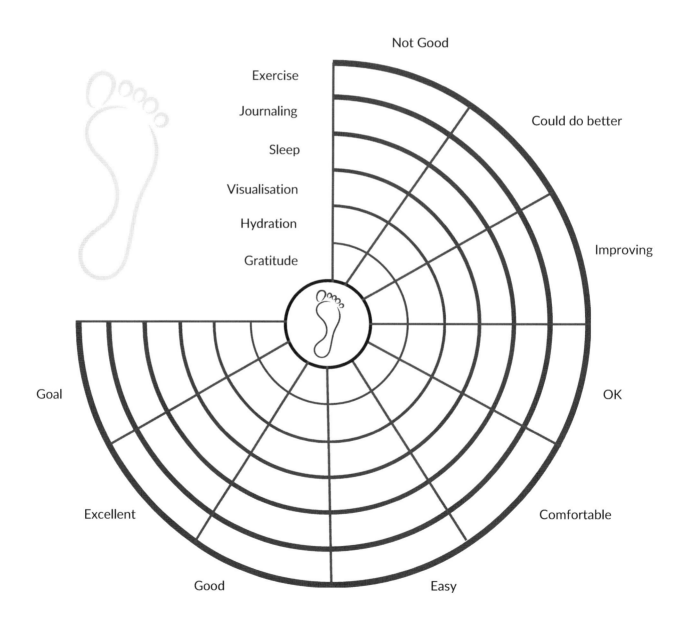

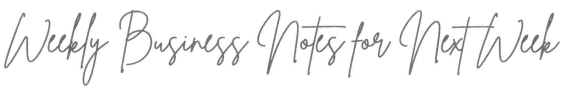

Weekly Business Notes for Next Week

Month:

Week:

Weekly Business Intentions

I must achieve this week:

1. ....

2. ....

3. ....

4. ....

5. ....

How many followers do you have:

Facebook Page: ....

Facebook Group: ....

Instagram: ....

LinkedIn: ....

Affirmation:

I will achieve and focus on my Intentions

Numbers:

What is my Financial Goal for the week?

How many clients would you like to see?   How many new clients would you like to see?

How will you achieve the numbers above:

....

....

....

Theme for the Week:

What subjects can you break your theme into subjects:

Monday:

Tuesday:

Wednesday:

Thursday:

Friday:

Weekend:

Social Media Locations:

Colour in the hearts when the content is posted or scheduled

	M	T	W	T	F	S	S
Facebook Page	♡	♡	♡	♡	♡	♡	♡
Facebook Group	♡	♡	♡	♡	♡	♡	♡
Facebook Live	♡	♡	♡	♡	♡	♡	♡
Instagram	♡	♡	♡	♡	♡	♡	♡
Instagram Stories	♡	♡	♡	♡	♡	♡	♡
LinkedIn	♡	♡	♡	♡	♡	♡	♡
Twitter	♡	♡	♡	♡	♡	♡	♡
Google	♡	♡	♡	♡	♡	♡	♡

Theme for the week Hashtags:

Month:

Week:

Selfcare Checks:

Colour in the hearts when you have achieved each self care step.

Colour in one for once and both for more than once.

Have you:

Exercised ♡ ♡

Journaled ♡ ♡

Affirmed your Affirmation ♡ ♡

5 minutes Silence ♡ ♡

Visualised where you want to be by the end of the week ♡ ♡

Written down 5 things a day you are grateful for ♡ ♡

Meditation ♡ ♡

Set my Intentions for the week ♡ ♡

Read a book ♡ ♡

I am grateful for:

1.

2.

3.

4.

5.

What will you do to celebrate the week?

What is your ONE selfcare non negotiable this week?

What was your unexpected WIN of the week?

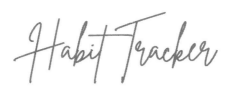

Habit Tracker

Habit trackers are exactly what they say they are. Map out your footsteps to keeping your new habits on track:

Where are you now?

Colour in how well you are doing today

This wheel is the start of your footsteps to creating some great habits to help you keep your business on sturdy footings.

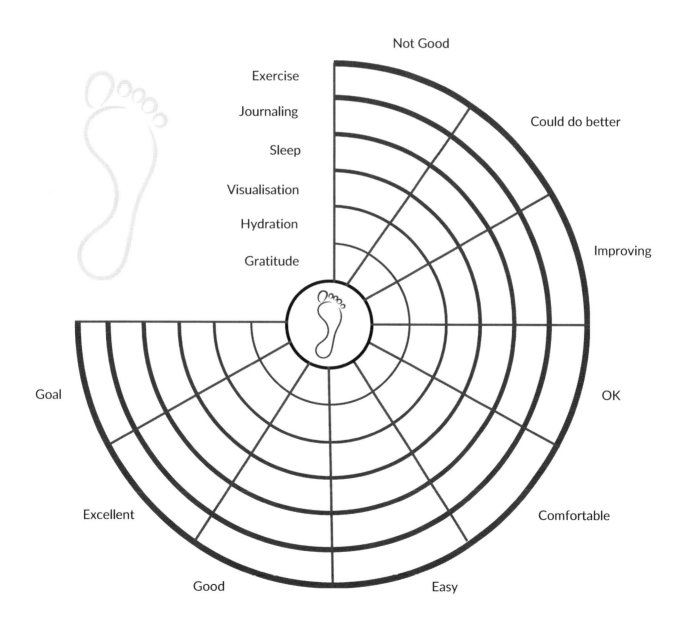

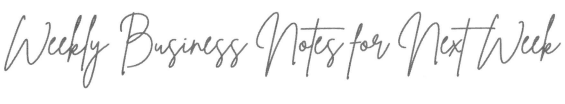

Weekly Business Notes for Next Week

Month:

Week:

I must achieve this week:

1. ....

2. ....

3. ....

4. ....

5. ....

How many followers do you have:

Facebook Page: ....

Facebook Group: ....

Instagram: ....

LinkedIn: ....

Affirmation:

Every day I have more reasons to smile and be happy

Numbers:

What is my Financial Goal for the week?

How many clients would you like to see?   How many new clients would you like to see?

How will you achieve the numbers above:

....

....

....

Theme for the Week:

Weekly Social Media Planning

What subjects can you break your theme into subjects:

Monday:

Tuesday:

Wednesday:

Thursday:

Friday:

Weekend:

Social Media Locations:

Colour in the hearts when the content is posted or scheduled

	M	T	W	T	F	S	S
Facebook Page	♡	♡	♡	♡	♡	♡	♡
Facebook Group	♡	♡	♡	♡	♡	♡	♡
Facebook Live	♡	♡	♡	♡	♡	♡	♡
Instagram	♡	♡	♡	♡	♡	♡	♡
Instagram Stories	♡	♡	♡	♡	♡	♡	♡
LinkedIn	♡	♡	♡	♡	♡	♡	♡
Twitter	♡	♡	♡	♡	♡	♡	♡
Google	♡	♡	♡	♡	♡	♡	♡

Theme for the week Hashtags:

Month:

Week:

Selfcare Checks:

Colour in the hearts when you have achieved each self care step.

Colour in one for once and both for more than once.

Have you:

Exercised ♡ ♡

Journaled ♡ ♡

Affirmed your Affirmation ♡ ♡

5 minutes Silence ♡ ♡

Visualised where you want to be by the end of the week ♡ ♡

Written down 5 things a day you are grateful for ♡ ♡

Meditation ♡ ♡

Set my Intentions for the week ♡ ♡

Read a book ♡ ♡

I am grateful for:

1.

2.

3.

4.

5.

What will you do to celebrate the week?

What is your ONE selfcare non negotiable this week?

What was your unexpected WIN of the week?

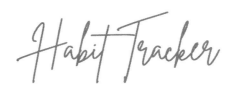

Habit Tracker

Habit trackers are exactly what they say they are. Map out your footsteps to keeping your new habits on track:

Where are you now?

Colour in how well you are doing today

This wheel is the start of your footsteps to creating some great habits to help you keep your business on sturdy footings.

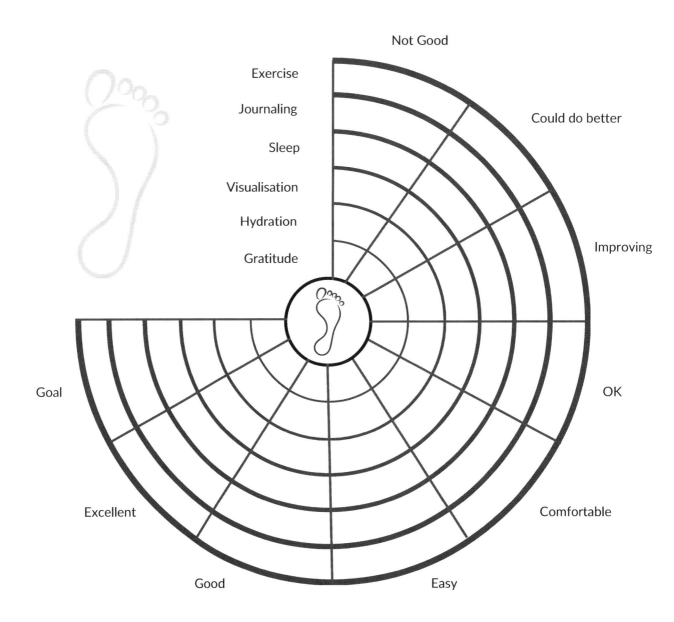

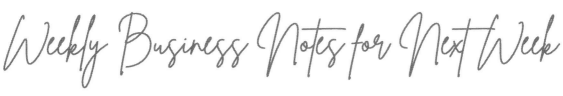

Weekly Business Notes for Next Week

Month:

Week:

I must achieve this week:

1. ....

2. ....

3. ....

4. ....

5. ....

How many followers do you have:

Facebook Page: ....

Facebook Group: ....

Instagram: ....

LinkedIn: ....

Affirmation:

I believe in myself
Be your No 1
cheerleader

Numbers:

What is my Financial Goal for the week?

How many clients would you like to see?   How many new clients would you like to see?

How will you achieve the numbers above:

....

....

....

Theme for the Week:

Weekly Social Media Planning

What subjects can you break your theme into subjects:

Monday:

Tuesday:

Wednesday:

Thursday:

Friday:

Weekend:

Social Media Locations:

Colour in the hearts when the content is posted or scheduled

	M	T	W	T	F	S	S
Facebook Page	♡	♡	♡	♡	♡	♡	♡
Facebook Group	♡	♡	♡	♡	♡	♡	♡
Facebook Live	♡	♡	♡	♡	♡	♡	♡
Instagram	♡	♡	♡	♡	♡	♡	♡
Instagram Stories	♡	♡	♡	♡	♡	♡	♡
LinkedIn	♡	♡	♡	♡	♡	♡	♡
Twitter	♡	♡	♡	♡	♡	♡	♡
Google	♡	♡	♡	♡	♡	♡	♡

Theme for the week Hashtags:

Month:

Week:

Selfcare Checks:

Colour in the hearts when you have achieved each self care step.

Colour in one for once and both for more than once.

Have you:

Exercised ♡ ♡

Journaled ♡ ♡

Affirmed your Affirmation ♡ ♡

5 minutes Silence ♡ ♡

Visualised where you want to be by the end of the week ♡ ♡

Written down 5 things a day you are grateful for ♡ ♡

Meditation ♡ ♡

Set my Intentions for the week ♡ ♡

Read a book ♡ ♡

I am grateful for:

1.

2.

3.

4.

5.

What will you do to celebrate the week?

What is your ONE selfcare non negotiable this week?

What was your unexpected WIN of the week?

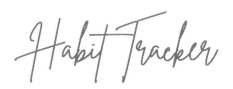

Habit Tracker

Habit trackers are exactly what they say they are. Map out your footsteps to keeping your new habits on track:

Where are you now?

Colour in how well you are doing today

This wheel is the start of your footsteps to creating some great habits to help you keep your business on sturdy footings.

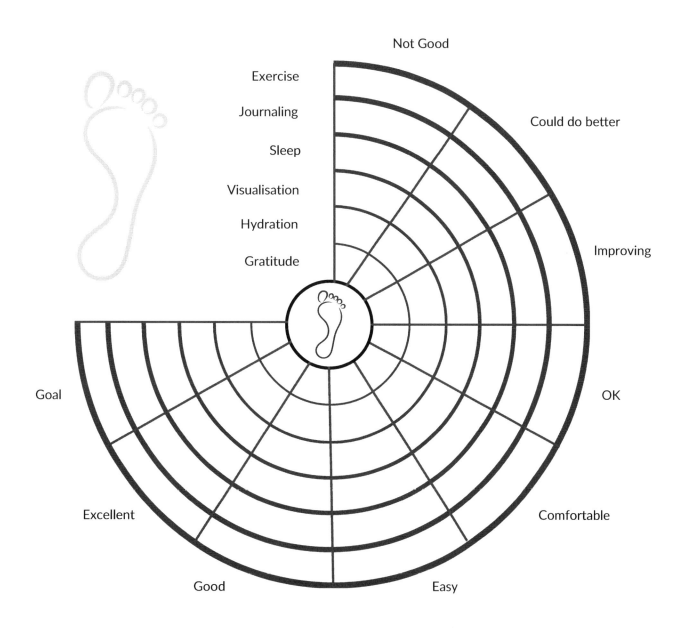

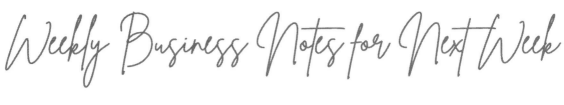

Weekly Business Notes for Next Week

Month:

Week:

Weekly Business Intentions

I must achieve this week:

1. ....

2. ....

3. ....

4. ....

5. ....

How many followers do you have:

Facebook Page: ....

Facebook Group: ....

Instagram: ....

LinkedIn: ....

Affirmation:

Every day I have more reasons to smile and be happy

Numbers:

What is my Financial Goal for the week?

How many clients would you like to see?   How many new clients would you like to see?

How will you achieve the numbers above:

....

....

....

Theme for the Week:

What subjects can you break your theme into subjects:

Monday:

Tuesday:

Wednesday:

Thursday:

Friday:

Weekend:

Social Media Locations:

Colour in the hearts when the content is posted or scheduled

Theme for the week Hashtags:

	M	T	W	T	F	S	S
Facebook Page	♡	♡	♡	♡	♡	♡	♡
Facebook Group	♡	♡	♡	♡	♡	♡	♡
Facebook Live	♡	♡	♡	♡	♡	♡	♡
Instagram	♡	♡	♡	♡	♡	♡	♡
Instagram Stories	♡	♡	♡	♡	♡	♡	♡
LinkedIn	♡	♡	♡	♡	♡	♡	♡
Twitter	♡	♡	♡	♡	♡	♡	♡
Google	♡	♡	♡	♡	♡	♡	♡

Month:

Week:

Selfcare Checks:

Colour in the hearts when you have achieved each self care step.

Colour in one for once and both for more than once.

Have you:

Exercised ♡ ♡

Journaled ♡ ♡

Affirmed your Affirmation ♡ ♡

5 minutes Silence ♡ ♡

Visualised where you want to be by the end of the week ♡ ♡

Written down 5 things a day you are grateful for ♡ ♡

Meditation ♡ ♡

Set my Intentions for the week ♡ ♡

Read a book ♡ ♡

I am grateful for:

1.

2.

3.

4.

5.

What will you do to celebrate the week?

What is your ONE selfcare non negotiable this week?

What was your unexpected WIN of the week?

Habit Tracker

Habit trackers are exactly what they say they are. Map out your footsteps to keeping your new habits on track:

Where are you now?

Colour in how well you are doing today

This wheel is the start of your footsteps to creating some great habits to help you keep your business on sturdy footings.

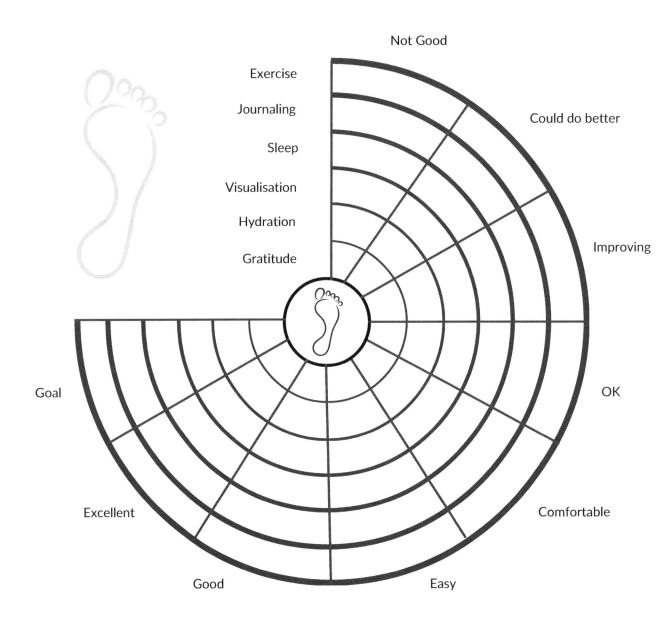

Month:

Week:

Monthly Checks:

Colour in the hearts when you have achieved each self care step.

Have you:

1. Updated your website ♡
2. Written a blog ♡
3. Read an inspirational book ♡
4. Gone "Live" on Facebook ♡
5. Done a "Reel" on Instagram ♡
6. Preschedule your posts for next month ♡
7. Planned your socials for next month ♡
8. Exercised each day/week ♡
9. Increased your Tax Savings Bank Account ♡
10. Booked a month end Celebration ♡
11. Paid all your invoices ♡
12. Are your accounts up to date ♡
13. Did your social media grow ♡
14. Did your client list grow ♡
15. Pay yourself ♡
16. Met up with a business colleague ♡
17. Attended a networking event ♡
18. Organised a treat for YOU ♡
19. Achieved your financial goals ♡
20. Increased your costs per client ♡

This month I am grateful for:

1.

2.

3.

4.

5.

What was your unexpected WIN of the month?

What will you do to celebrate next month?

Journal your Thoughts of the Month:

_____

_____

_____

_____

Month:
Prompts:
What was good,
What could I have improved on,
What have I enjoyed,
What questions do I need to ask,
Who can I connect with.

_____

_____

_____

_____

_____

_____

_____

_____

_____

_____

_____

_____

_____

_____

Journal your Thoughts of the Month:

My To Do List:

_____

_____

_____

_____

_____

_____

_____

_____

_____

_____

_____

_____

_____

_____

My Personal Affirmation for the month:

Date:

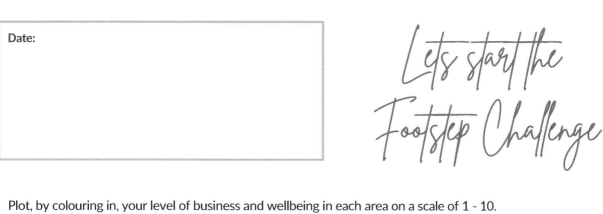

Plot, by colouring in, your level of business and wellbeing in each area on a scale of 1 - 10.
1 being the first foot and not so good and 10 being the last foot and top totch:

Personal Development - Training, Reading &
Learning

Exercise and Diet - Maybe Yoga, Pilates, Walking
or Running and the fuel you supply to your body to
enable you to be effective

Sleep - Napping or Sleeping

Finances, ie Accounts, Paying yourself etc

Social inc Networking & Business Interaction

Downtime - Time you spend with Family and Friends

Emotional Well Being

 Fun & Celebrating

Quarter :

Months included:

Quarterly Social Media Growth

	Facebook Page A	Facebook Group B	Instagram C	Total A+B+C	Growth on previous month
Week 1					0
Week 2					
Week 3					
Week 4					
Week 5					
Week 6					
Week 7					
Week 8					
Week 9					
Week 10					
Week 11					
Week 12					
TOTALS					

Quarter :

Months included:

Quarterly Clients & Turnover Growth

	No of Clients A	No of New Clients B	WeeklyTurnover C	Turnover per client C/A
Week 1				
Week 2				
Week 3				
Week 4				
Week 5				
Week 6				
Week 7				
Week 8				
Week 9				
Week 10				
Week 11				
Week 12				
TOTALS				

Journal your Thoughts of the Quarter:

_____

_____

_____

_____

Month:

Prompts in 3 moths time:

Where do you want to be

What do you want to have achieved

What do you want to learn

Do you need to research a course

My To Do List

BUSINESS:

_____
_____
_____
_____
_____
_____
_____
_____
_____
_____
_____
_____
_____

PERSONAL:

_____
_____
_____
_____
_____
_____
_____
_____
_____

Well Done

Month:

Week:

Weekly Business Intentions

I must achieve this week:

1. ....

2. ....

3. ....

4. ....

5. ....

How many followers do you have:

Facebook Page: ....

Facebook Group: ....

Instagram: ....

LinkedIn: ....

Affirmation:

Numbers:

What is my Financial Goal for the week?

How many clients would you like to see?   How many new clients would you like to see?

How will you achieve the numbers above:

....

....

....

Weekly Social Media Planning

Theme for the Week:

What subjects can you break your theme into subjects:

Monday:

Tuesday:

Wednesday:

Thursday:

Friday:

Weekend:

Social Media Locations:

Colour in the hearts when the content is posted or scheduled

	M	T	W	T	F	S	S
Facebook Page	♡	♡	♡	♡	♡	♡	♡
Facebook Group	♡	♡	♡	♡	♡	♡	♡
Facebook Live	♡	♡	♡	♡	♡	♡	♡
Instagram	♡	♡	♡	♡	♡	♡	♡
Instagram Stories	♡	♡	♡	♡	♡	♡	♡
LinkedIn	♡	♡	♡	♡	♡	♡	♡
Twitter	♡	♡	♡	♡	♡	♡	♡
Google	♡	♡	♡	♡	♡	♡	♡

Theme for the week Hashtags:

Month:

Week:

Selfcare Checks:

Colour in the hearts when you have achieved each self care step.

Colour in one for once and both for more than once.

Have you:

Exercised ♡ ♡

Journaled ♡ ♡

Affirmed your Affirmation ♡ ♡

5 minutes Silence ♡ ♡

Visualised where you want to be by the end of the week ♡ ♡

Written down 5 things a day you are grateful for ♡ ♡

Meditation ♡ ♡

Set my Intentions for the week ♡ ♡

Read a book ♡ ♡

I am grateful for:

1.

2.

3.

4.

5.

What will you do to celebrate the week?

What is your ONE selfcare non negotiable this week?

What was your unexpected WIN of the week?

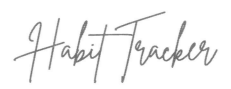

Habit Tracker

Habit trackers are exactly what they say they are. Map out your footsteps to keeping your new habits on track:

Where are you now?

Colour in how well you are doing today

This wheel is the start of your footsteps to creating some great habits to help you keep your business on sturdy footings.

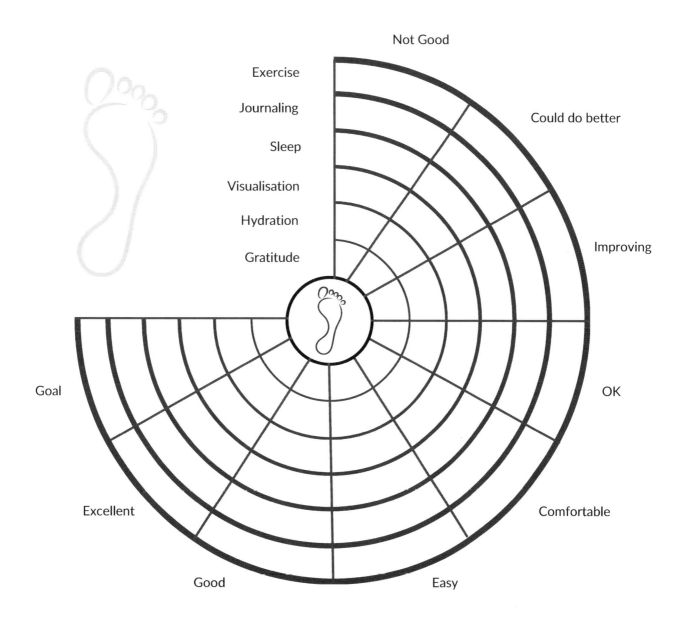

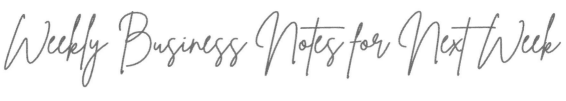

Weekly Business Notes for Next Week

Month:

Week:

Weekly Business Intentions

I must achieve this week:

1. ....

2. ....

3. ....

4. ....

5. ....

How many followers do you have:

Facebook Page: ....

Facebook Group: ....

Instagram: ....

LinkedIn: ....

Affirmation:

Numbers:

What is my Financial Goal for the week?

How many clients would you like to see?   How many new clients would you like to see?

How will you achieve the numbers above:

....

....

....

Theme for the Week:

Weekly Social Media Planning

What subjects can you break your theme into subjects:

Monday:

Tuesday:

Wednesday:

Thursday:

Friday:

Weekend:

Social Media Locations:

Colour in the hearts when the content is posted or scheduled

	M	T	W	T	F	S	S
Facebook Page	♡	♡	♡	♡	♡	♡	♡
Facebook Group	♡	♡	♡	♡	♡	♡	♡
Facebook Live	♡	♡	♡	♡	♡	♡	♡
Instagram	♡	♡	♡	♡	♡	♡	♡
Instagram Stories	♡	♡	♡	♡	♡	♡	♡
LinkedIn	♡	♡	♡	♡	♡	♡	♡
Twitter	♡	♡	♡	♡	♡	♡	♡
Google	♡	♡	♡	♡	♡	♡	♡

Theme for the week Hashtags:

Month:

Week:

Selfcare Checks:

Colour in the hearts when you have achieved each self care step.

Colour in one for once and both for more than once.

Have you:

Exercised	♡	♡
Journaled	♡	♡
Affirmed your Affirmation	♡	♡
5 minutes Silence	♡	♡
Visualised where you want to be by the end of the week	♡	♡
Written down 5 things a day you are grateful for	♡	♡
Meditation	♡	♡
Set my Intentions for the week	♡	♡
Read a book	♡	♡

I am grateful for:

1.

2.

3.

4.

5.

What will you do to celebrate the week?

What is your ONE selfcare non negotiable this week?

What was your unexpected WIN of the week?

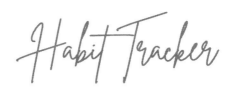

Habit Tracker

Habit trackers are exactly what they say they are. Map out your footsteps to keeping your new habits on track:

Where are you now?

Colour in how well you are doing today

This wheel is the start of your footsteps to creating some great habits to help you keep your business on sturdy footings.

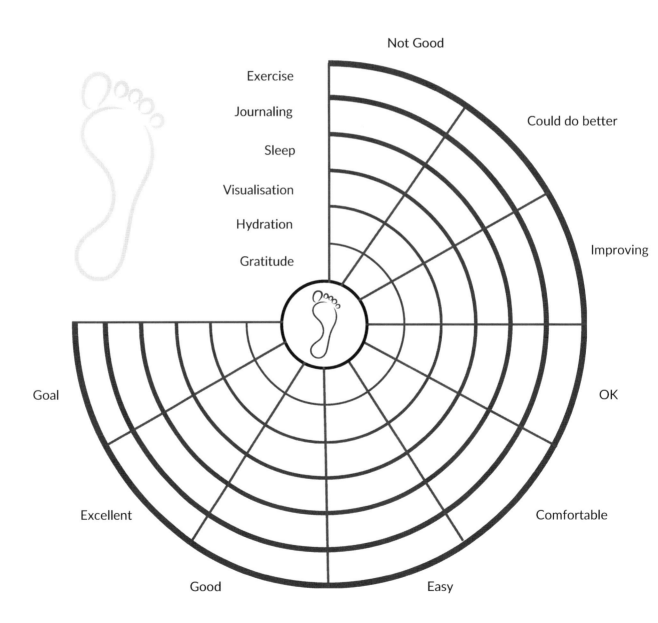

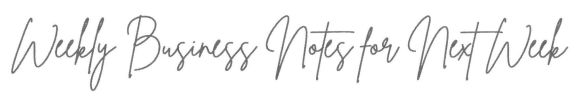

Weekly Business Notes for Next Week

Month:

Week:

Weekly Business Intentions

I must achieve this week:

1. ....

2. ....

3. ....

4. ....

5. ....

How many followers do you have:

Facebook Page: ....

Facebook Group: ....

Instagram: ....

LinkedIn: ....

Affirmation:

Numbers:

What is my Financial Goal for the week?

How many clients would you like to see?   How many new clients would you like to see?

How will you achieve the numbers above:

....

....

....

Theme for the Week:

What subjects can you break your theme into subjects:

Monday:

Tuesday:

Wednesday:

Thursday:

Friday:

Weekend:

Social Media Locations:

Colour in the hearts when the content is posted or scheduled

	M	T	W	T	F	S	S
Facebook Page	♡	♡	♡	♡	♡	♡	♡
Facebook Group	♡	♡	♡	♡	♡	♡	♡
Facebook Live	♡	♡	♡	♡	♡	♡	♡
Instagram	♡	♡	♡	♡	♡	♡	♡
Instagram Stories	♡	♡	♡	♡	♡	♡	♡
LinkedIn	♡	♡	♡	♡	♡	♡	♡
Twitter	♡	♡	♡	♡	♡	♡	♡
Google	♡	♡	♡	♡	♡	♡	♡

Theme for the week Hashtags:

Month:

Week:

Weekly Business Checks and Selfcare

Selfcare Checks:

Colour in the hearts when you have achieved each self care step.

Colour in one for once and both for more than once.

Have you:

Exercised

Journaled

Affirmed your Affirmation

5 minutes Silence

Visualised where you want to be by the end of the week

Written down 5 things a day you are grateful for

Meditation

Set my Intentions for the week

Read a book

I am grateful for:

1.

2.

3.

4.

5.

What will you do to celebrate the week?

What is your ONE selfcare non negotiable this week?

What was your unexpected WIN of the week?

Habit Tracker

Habit trackers are exactly what they say they are. Map out your footsteps to keeping your new habits on track:

Where are you now?

Colour in how well you are doing today

This wheel is the start of your footsteps to creating some great habits to help you keep your business on sturdy footings.

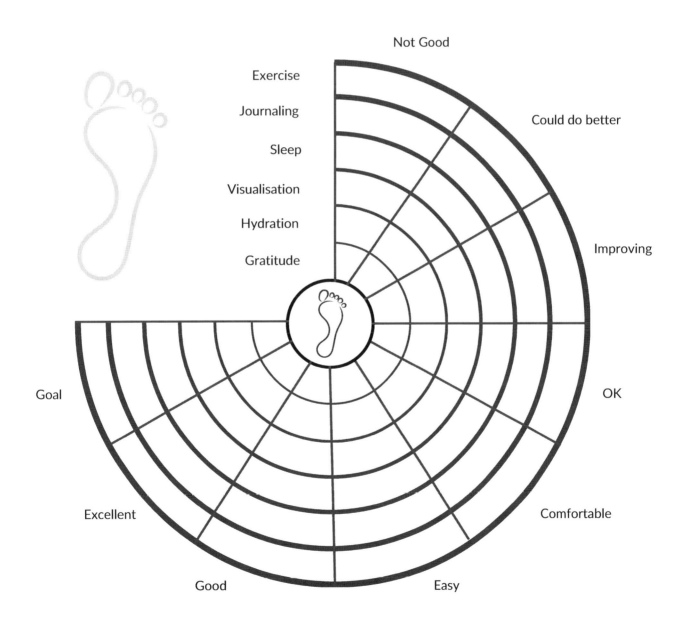

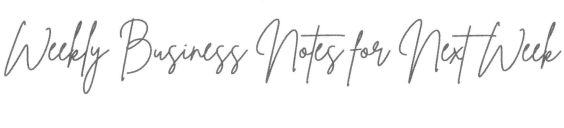

Weekly Business Notes for Next Week

Month:

Week:

Weekly Business Intentions

I must achieve this week:

1. ....
2. ....
3. ....
4. ....
5. ....

How many followers do you have:

Facebook Page: ....

Facebook Group: ....

Instagram: ....

LinkedIn: ....

Affirmation:

Numbers:

What is my Financial Goal for the week?

How many clients would you like to see?   How many new clients would you like to see?

How will you achieve the numbers above:

....

....

....

Theme for the Week:

What subjects can you break your theme into subjects:

Monday:

Tuesday:

Wednesday:

Thursday:

Friday:

Weekend:

Social Media Locations:

Colour in the hearts when the content is posted or scheduled

	M	T	W	T	F	S	S
Facebook Page	♡	♡	♡	♡	♡	♡	♡
Facebook Group	♡	♡	♡	♡	♡	♡	♡
Facebook Live	♡	♡	♡	♡	♡	♡	♡
Instagram	♡	♡	♡	♡	♡	♡	♡
Instagram Stories	♡	♡	♡	♡	♡	♡	♡
LinkedIn	♡	♡	♡	♡	♡	♡	♡
Twitter	♡	♡	♡	♡	♡	♡	♡
Google	♡	♡	♡	♡	♡	♡	♡

Theme for the week Hashtags:

Month:

Week:

Selfcare Checks:

Colour in the hearts when you have achieved each self care step.

Colour in one for once and both for more than once.

Have you:

Exercised ♡ ♡

Journaled ♡ ♡

Affirmed your Affirmation ♡ ♡

5 minutes Silence ♡ ♡

Visualised where you want to be by the end of the week ♡ ♡

Written down 5 things a day you are grateful for ♡ ♡

Meditation ♡ ♡

Set my Intentions for the week ♡ ♡

Read a book ♡ ♡

I am grateful for:

1.

2.

3.

4.

5.

What will you do to celebrate the week?

What is your ONE selfcare non negotiable this week?

What was your unexpected WIN of the week?

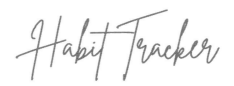

Habit Tracker

Habit trackers are exactly what they say they are. Map out your footsteps to keeping your new habits on track:

Where are you now?

Colour in how well you are doing today

This wheel is the start of your footsteps to creating some great habits to help you keep your business on sturdy footings.

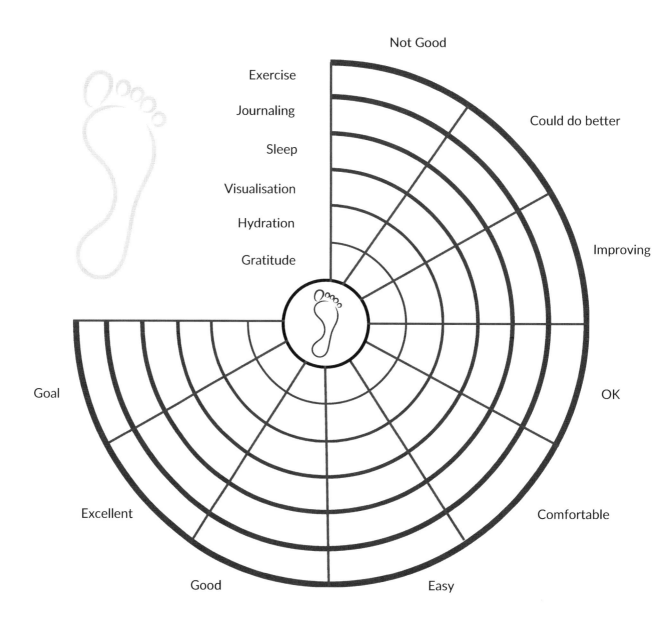

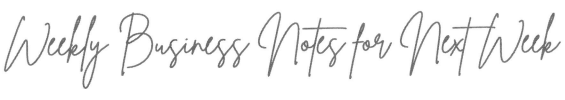

Weekly Business Notes for Next Week

Month:

Week:

Weekly Business Intentions

I must achieve this week:

1. ....

2. ....

3. ....

4. ....

5. ....

How many followers do you have:

Facebook Page: ....

Facebook Group: ....

Instagram: ....

LinkedIn: ....

Affirmation:

Numbers:

What is my Financial Goal for the week?

How many clients would you like to see?   How many new clients would you like to see?

How will you achieve the numbers above:

....

....

....

Theme for the Week:

Weekly Social Media Planning

What subjects can you break your theme into subjects:

Monday:

Tuesday:

Wednesday:

Thursday:

Friday:

Weekend:

Social Media Locations:

Colour in the hearts when the content is posted or scheduled

	M	T	W	T	F	S	S
Facebook Page	♡	♡	♡	♡	♡	♡	♡
Facebook Group	♡	♡	♡	♡	♡	♡	♡
Facebook Live	♡	♡	♡	♡	♡	♡	♡
Instagram	♡	♡	♡	♡	♡	♡	♡
Instagram Stories	♡	♡	♡	♡	♡	♡	♡
LinkedIn	♡	♡	♡	♡	♡	♡	♡
Twitter	♡	♡	♡	♡	♡	♡	♡
Google	♡	♡	♡	♡	♡	♡	♡

Theme for the week Hashtags:

Month:

Week:

Selfcare Checks:

Colour in the hearts when you have achieved each self care step.

Colour in one for once and both for more than once.

Have you:

Exercised

Journaled

Affirmed your Affirmation

5 minutes Silence

Visualised where you want to be by the end of the week

Written down 5 things a day you are grateful for

Meditation

Set my Intentions for the week

Read a book

I am grateful for:

1.

2.

3.

4.

5.

What will you do to celebrate the week?

What is your ONE selfcare non negotiable this week?

What was your unexpected WIN of the week?

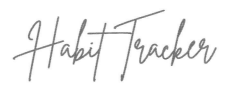

Habit Tracker

Habit trackers are exactly what they say they are. Map out your footsteps to keeping your new habits on track:

Where are you now?

Colour in how well you are doing today

This wheel is the start of your footsteps to creating some great habits to help you keep your business on sturdy footings.

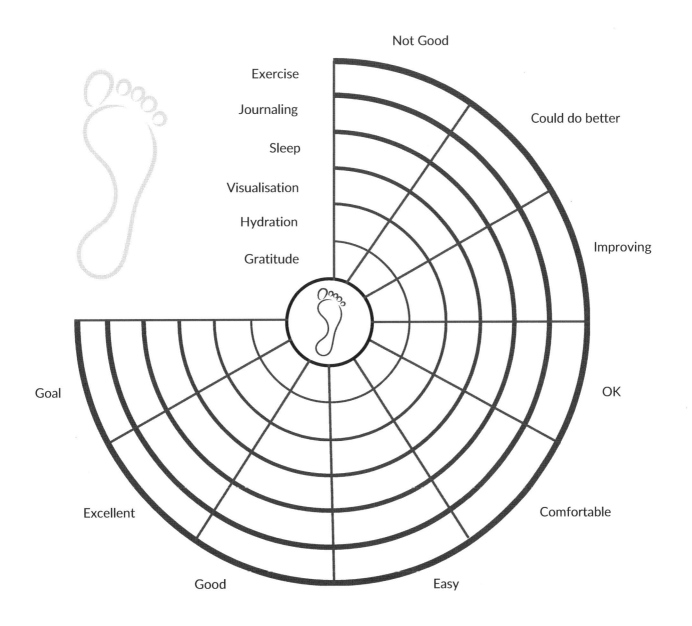

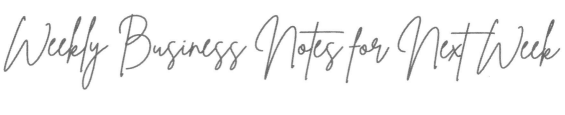

Weekly Business Notes for Next Week

| Month: | _Monthly Business_ |
| Week: | _Checks Up_ |

Monthly Checks:

Colour in the hearts when you have achieved each self care step.

Have you:

1. Updated your website ♡
2. Written a blog ♡
3. Read an inspirational book ♡
4. Gone "Live" on Facebook ♡
5. Done a "Reel" on Instagram ♡
6. Preschedule your posts for next month ♡
7. Planned your socials for next month ♡
8. Exercised each day/week ♡
9. Increased your Tax Savings Bank Account ♡
10. Booked a month end Celebration ♡
11. Paid all your invoices ♡
12. Are your accounts up to date ♡
13. Did your social media grow ♡
14. Did your client list grow ♡
15. Pay yourself ♡
16. Met up with a business colleague ♡
17. Attended a networking event ♡
18. Organised a treat for YOU ♡
19. Achieved your financial goals ♡
20. Increased your costs per client ♡

This month I am grateful for:

1.

2.

3.

4.

5.

What was your unexpected WIN of the month?

What will you do to celebrate next month?

Journal your Thoughts of the Month:

Month:

Prompts:

What was good,
What could I have improved on,
What have I enjoyed,
What questions do I need to ask,
Who can I connect with.

Journal your Thoughts of the Month:

_____

_____

_____

_____

_____

_____

_____

_____

_____

_____

_____

_____

_____

_____

_____

_____

_____

_____

_____

_____

_____

My To Do List:

_____

_____

_____

_____

_____

_____

_____

_____

_____

_____

_____

_____

My Personal Affirmation for the month:

Date:

Lets Re Do the Footstep Challenge

Plot by colouring in your level of business and wellbeing in each area on a scale of 1 - 10 (1 being the first foot) considering the following:

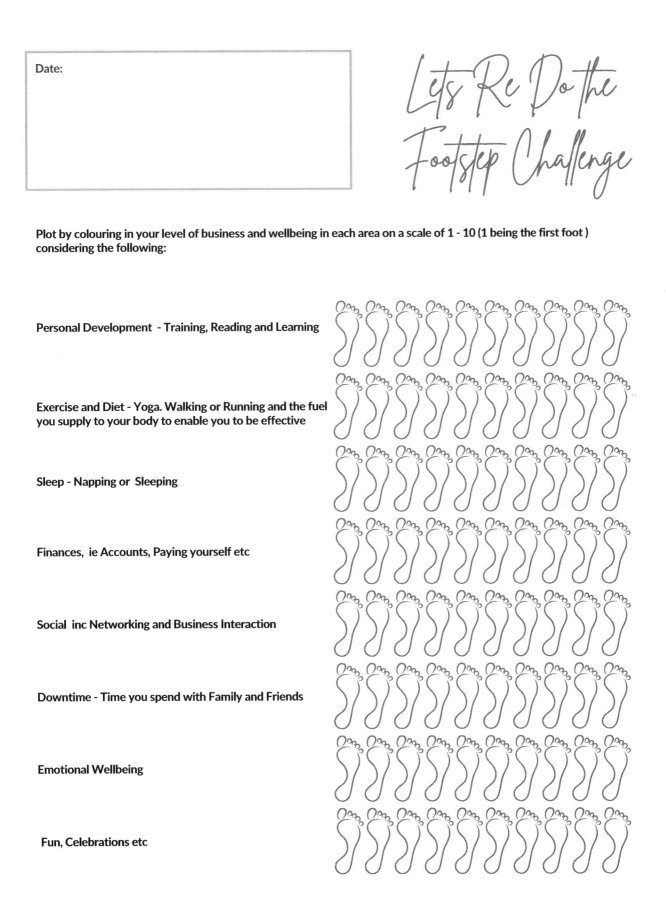

Personal Development - Training, Reading and Learning

Exercise and Diet - Yoga. Walking or Running and the fuel you supply to your body to enable you to be effective

Sleep - Napping or Sleeping

Finances, ie Accounts, Paying yourself etc

Social inc Networking and Business Interaction

Downtime - Time you spend with Family and Friends

Emotional Wellbeing

Fun, Celebrations etc

Month:

Week:

Weekly Business Intentions

I must achieve this week:

1. ....
2. ....
3. ....
4. ....
5. ....

How many followers do you have:

Facebook Page: ....

Facebook Group: ....

Instagram: ....

LinkedIn: ....

Affirmation:

Numbers:

What is my Financial Goal for the week?

How many clients would you like to see?   How many new clients would you like to see?

How will you achieve the numbers above:

....

....

....

Theme for the Week:

Weekly Social Media Planning

What subjects can you break your theme into subjects:

Monday:

Tuesday:

Wednesday:

Thursday:

Friday:

Weekend:

Social Media Locations:

Colour in the hearts when the content is posted or scheduled

	M	T	W	T	F	S	S
Facebook Page	♡	♡	♡	♡	♡	♡	♡
Facebook Group	♡	♡	♡	♡	♡	♡	♡
Facebook Live	♡	♡	♡	♡	♡	♡	♡
Instagram	♡	♡	♡	♡	♡	♡	♡
Instagram Stories	♡	♡	♡	♡	♡	♡	♡
LinkedIn	♡	♡	♡	♡	♡	♡	♡
Twitter	♡	♡	♡	♡	♡	♡	♡
Google	♡	♡	♡	♡	♡	♡	♡

Theme for the week Hashtags:

Month:	
Week:	

Selfcare Checks:

Colour in the hearts when you have achieved each self care step.

Colour in one for once and both for more than once.

Have you:

Exercised ♡ ♡

Journaled ♡ ♡

Affirmed your Affirmation ♡ ♡

5 minutes Silence ♡ ♡

Visualised where you want to be by the end of the week ♡ ♡

Written down 5 things a day you are grateful for ♡ ♡

Meditation ♡ ♡

Set my Intentions for the week ♡ ♡

Read a book ♡ ♡

I am grateful for:

1.

2.

3.

4.

5.

What will you do to celebrate the week?

What is your ONE selfcare non negotiable this week?

What was your unexpected WIN of the week?

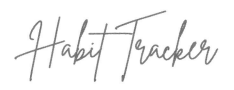

Habit Tracker

Habit trackers are exactly what they say they are. Map out your footsteps to keeping your new habits on track:

Where are you now?

Colour in how well you are doing today

This wheel is the start of your footsteps to creating some great habits to help you keep your business on sturdy footings.

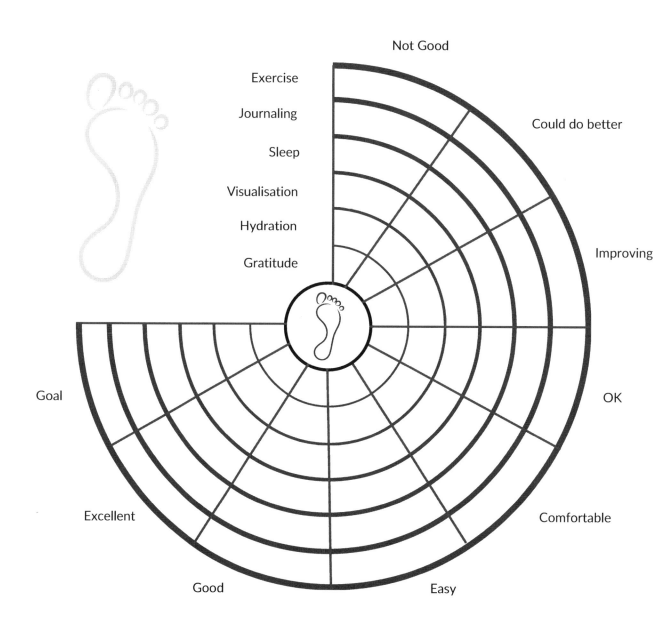

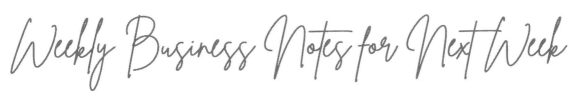

Weekly Business Notes for Next Week

Month:

Week:

Weekly Business Intentions

I must achieve this week:

1. ....

2. ....

3. ....

4. ....

5. ....

How many followers do you have:

Facebook Page: ....

Facebook Group: ....

Instagram: ....

LinkedIn: ....

Affirmation:

Numbers:

What is my Financial Goal for the week?

How many clients would you like to see?   How many new clients would you like to see?

How will you achieve the numbers above:

....

....

....

Theme for the Week:

Weekly Social Media Planning

What subjects can you break your theme into subjects:

Monday:

Tuesday:

Wednesday:

Thursday:

Friday:

Weekend:

Social Media Locations:

Colour in the hearts when the content is posted or scheduled

	M	T	W	T	F	S	S
Facebook Page	♡	♡	♡	♡	♡	♡	♡
Facebook Group	♡	♡	♡	♡	♡	♡	♡
Facebook Live	♡	♡	♡	♡	♡	♡	♡
Instagram	♡	♡	♡	♡	♡	♡	♡
Instagram Stories	♡	♡	♡	♡	♡	♡	♡
LinkedIn	♡	♡	♡	♡	♡	♡	♡
Twitter	♡	♡	♡	♡	♡	♡	♡
Google	♡	♡	♡	♡	♡	♡	♡

Theme for the week Hashtags:

Month:

Week:

Selfcare Checks:

Colour in the hearts when you have achieved each self care step.

Colour in one for once and both for more than once.

Have you:

Exercised ♡ ♡

Journaled ♡ ♡

Affirmed your Affirmation ♡ ♡

5 minutes Silence ♡ ♡

Visualised where you want to be by the end of the week ♡ ♡

Written down 5 things a day you are grateful for ♡ ♡

Meditation ♡ ♡

Set my Intentions for the week ♡ ♡

Read a book ♡ ♡

I am grateful for:

1.

2.

3.

4.

5.

What will you do to celebrate the week?

What is your ONE selfcare non negotiable this week?

What was your unexpected WIN of the week?

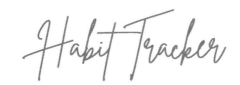

Habit Tracker

Habit trackers are exactly what they say they are. Map out your footsteps to keeping your new habits on track:

Where are you now?

Colour in how well you are doing today

This wheel is the start of your footsteps to creating some great habits to help you keep your business on sturdy footings.

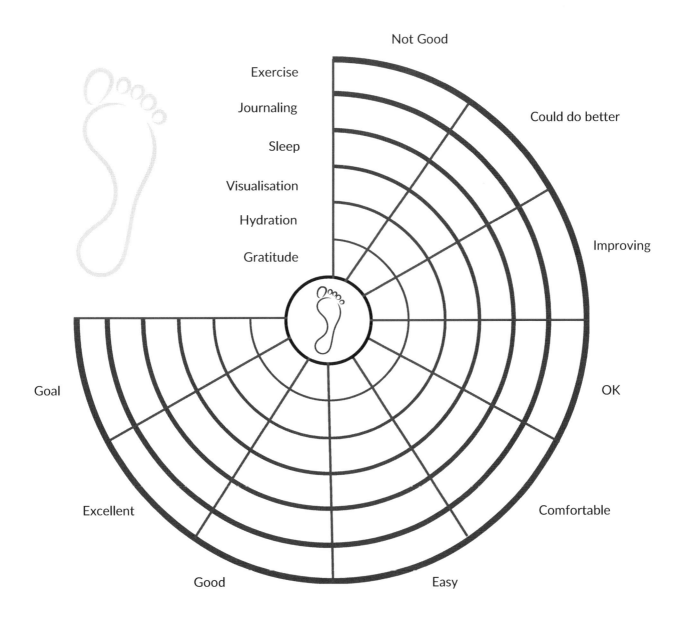

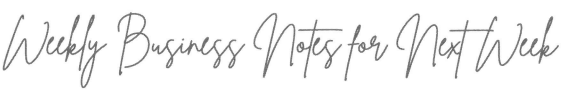

Weekly Business Notes for Next Week

Month:

Week:

Weekly Business Intentions

I must achieve this week:

1. ....

2. ....

3. ....

4. ....

5. ....

How many followers do you have:

Facebook Page: ....

Facebook Group: ....

Instagram: ....

LinkedIn: ....

Affirmation:

Numbers:

What is my Financial Goal for the week?

How many clients would you like to see?   How many new clients would you like to see?

How will you achieve the numbers above:

....

....

....

Theme for the Week:

Weekly Social Media Planning

What subjects can you break your theme into subjects:

Monday:

Tuesday:

Wednesday:

Thursday:

Friday:

Weekend:

Social Media Locations:

Colour in the hearts when the content is posted or scheduled

	M	T	W	T	F	S	S
Facebook Page	♡	♡	♡	♡	♡	♡	♡
Facebook Group	♡	♡	♡	♡	♡	♡	♡
Facebook Live	♡	♡	♡	♡	♡	♡	♡
Instagram	♡	♡	♡	♡	♡	♡	♡
Instagram Stories	♡	♡	♡	♡	♡	♡	♡
LinkedIn	♡	♡	♡	♡	♡	♡	♡
Twitter	♡	♡	♡	♡	♡	♡	♡
Google	♡	♡	♡	♡	♡	♡	♡

Theme for the week Hashtags:

Month:

Week:

Weekly Business
Checks and Selfcare

Selfcare Checks:

Colour in the hearts when you have achieved each self care step.

Colour in one for once and both for more than once.

Have you:

Exercised ♡ ♡

Journaled ♡ ♡

Affirmed your Affirmation ♡ ♡

5 minutes Silence ♡ ♡

Visualised where you want to be by the end of the week ♡ ♡

Written down 5 things a day you are grateful for ♡ ♡

Meditation ♡ ♡

Set my Intentions for the week ♡ ♡

Read a book ♡ ♡

I am grateful for:

1.

2.

3.

4.

5.

What will you do to celebrate the week?

What is your ONE selfcare non negotiable this week?

What was your unexpected WIN of the week?

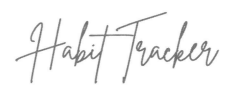

Habit Tracker

Habit trackers are exactly what they say they are. Map out your footsteps to keeping your new habits on track:

Where are you now?

Colour in how well you are doing today

This wheel is the start of your footsteps to creating some great habits to help you keep your business on sturdy footings.

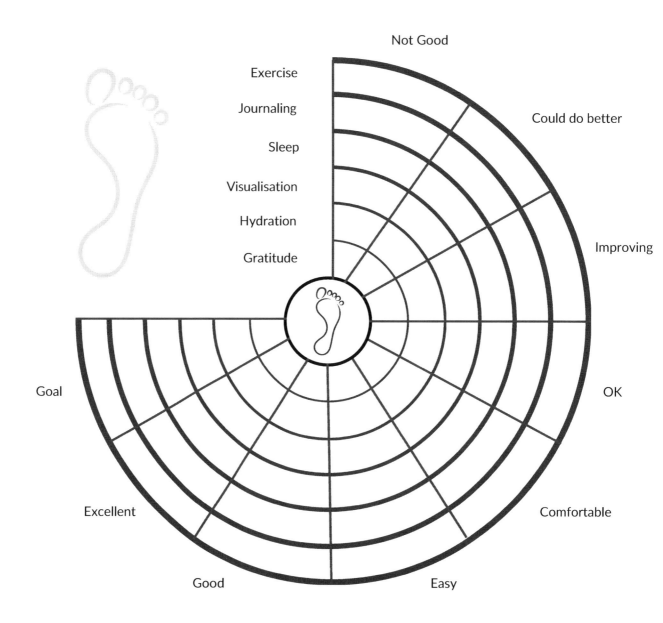

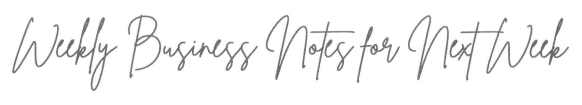

Weekly Business Notes for Next Week

Month:

Week:

Weekly Business Intentions

I must achieve this week:

1. ....

2. ....

3. ....

4. ....

5. ....

How many followers do you have:

Facebook Page: ....

Facebook Group: ....

Instagram: ....

LinkedIn: ....

Affirmation:

Numbers:

What is my Financial Goal for the week?

How many clients would you like to see?   How many new clients would you like to see?

How will you achieve the numbers above:

....

....

....

Theme for the Week:

Weekly Social Media Planning

What subjects can you break your theme into subjects:

Monday:

Tuesday:

Wednesday:

Thursday:

Friday:

Weekend:

Social Media Locations:

Colour in the hearts when the content is posted or scheduled

	M	T	W	T	F	S	S
Facebook Page	♡	♡	♡	♡	♡	♡	♡
Facebook Group	♡	♡	♡	♡	♡	♡	♡
Facebook Live	♡	♡	♡	♡	♡	♡	♡
Instagram	♡	♡	♡	♡	♡	♡	♡
Instagram Stories	♡	♡	♡	♡	♡	♡	♡
LinkedIn	♡	♡	♡	♡	♡	♡	♡
Twitter	♡	♡	♡	♡	♡	♡	♡
Google	♡	♡	♡	♡	♡	♡	♡

Theme for the week Hashtags:

Month:

Week:

Selfcare Checks:

Colour in the hearts when you have achieved each self care step.

Colour in one for once and both for more than once.

Have you:

Exercised ♡ ♡

Journaled ♡ ♡

Affirmed your Affirmation ♡ ♡

5 minutes Silence ♡ ♡

Visualised where you want to be by the end of the week ♡ ♡

Written down 5 things a day you are grateful for ♡ ♡

Meditation ♡ ♡

Set my Intentions for the week ♡ ♡

Read a book ♡ ♡

I am grateful for:

1.

2.

3.

4.

5.

What will you do to celebrate the week?

What is your ONE selfcare non negotiable this week?

What was your unexpected WIN of the week?

Habit Tracker

Habit trackers are exactly what they say they are. Map out your footsteps to keeping your new habits on track:

Where are you now?

Colour in how well you are doing today

This wheel is the start of your footsteps to creating some great habits to help you keep your business on sturdy footings.

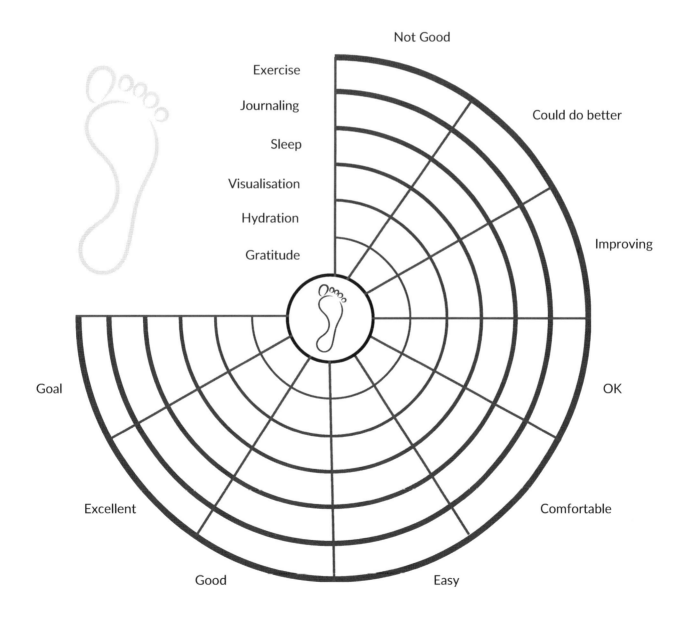

Month:

Week:

Weekly Business Intentions

I must achieve this week:

1. ....

2. ....

3. ....

4. ....

5. ....

How many followers do you have:

Facebook Page: ....

Facebook Group: ....

Instagram: ....

LinkedIn: ....

Affirmation:

Numbers:

What is my Financial Goal for the week?

How many clients would you like to see?   How many new clients would you like to see?

How will you achieve the numbers above:

....

....

....

Theme for the Week:

Weekly Social Media Planning

What subjects can you break your theme into subjects:

Monday:

Tuesday:

Wednesday:

Thursday:

Friday:

Weekend:

Social Media Locations:

Colour in the hearts when the content is posted or scheduled

	M	T	W	T	F	S	S
Facebook Page	♡	♡	♡	♡	♡	♡	♡
Facebook Group	♡	♡	♡	♡	♡	♡	♡
Facebook Live	♡	♡	♡	♡	♡	♡	♡
Instagram	♡	♡	♡	♡	♡	♡	♡
Instagram Stories	♡	♡	♡	♡	♡	♡	♡
LinkedIn	♡	♡	♡	♡	♡	♡	♡
Twitter	♡	♡	♡	♡	♡	♡	♡
Google	♡	♡	♡	♡	♡	♡	♡

Theme for the week Hashtags:

Month:

Week:

Selfcare Checks:

Colour in the hearts when you have achieved each self care step.

Colour in one for once and both for more than once.

Have you:

Exercised ♡ ♡

Journaled ♡ ♡

Affirmed your Affirmation ♡ ♡

5 minutes Silence ♡ ♡

Visualised where you want to be by the end of the week ♡ ♡

Written down 5 things a day you are grateful for ♡ ♡

Meditation ♡ ♡

Set my Intentions for the week ♡ ♡

Read a book ♡ ♡

I am grateful for:

1.

2.

3.

4.

5.

What will you do to celebrate the week?

What is your ONE selfcare non negotiable this week?

What was your unexpected WIN of the week?

Habit Tracker

Habit trackers are exactly what they say they are. Map out your footsteps to keeping your new habits on track:

Where are you now?

Colour in how well you are doing today

This wheel is the start of your footsteps to creating some great habits to help you keep your business on sturdy footings.

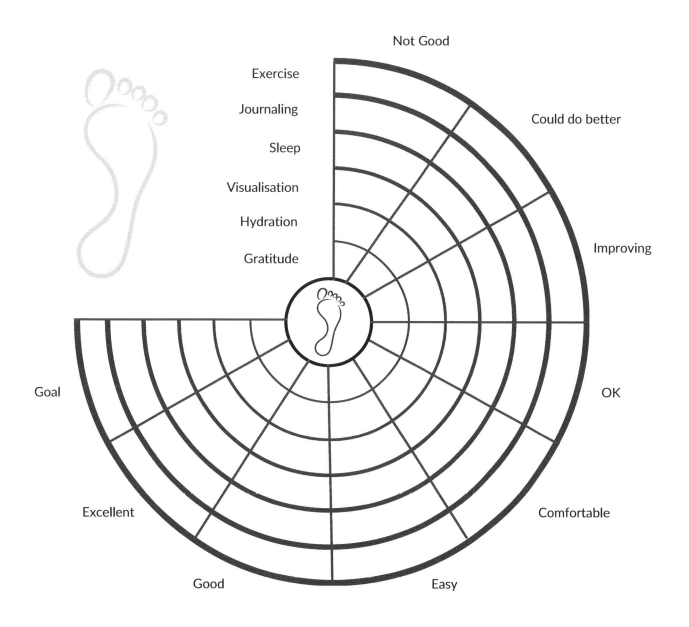

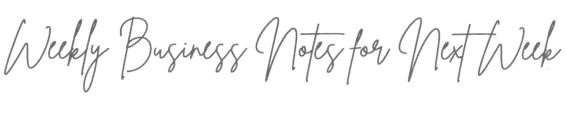

Weekly Business Notes for Next Week

Month:

Week:

Monthly Business Checks Up

Monthly Checks:

Colour in the hearts when you have achieved each self care step.

Have you:

1. Updated your website ♡
2. Written a blog ♡
3. Read an inspirational book ♡
4. Gone "Live" on Facebook ♡
5. Done a "Reel" on Instagram ♡
6. Preschedule your posts for next month ♡
7. Planned your socials for next month ♡
8. Exercised each day/week ♡
9. Increased your Tax Savings Bank Account ♡
10. Booked a month end Celebration ♡
11. Paid all your invoices ♡
12. Are your accounts up to date ♡
13. Did your social media grow ♡
14. Did your client list grow ♡
15. Pay yourself ♡
16. Met up with a business colleague ♡
17. Attended a networking event ♡
18. Organised a treat for YOU ♡
19. Achieved your financial goals ♡
20. Increased your costs per client ♡

This month I am grateful for:

1.

2.

3.

4.

5.

What was your unexpected WIN of the month?

What will you do to celebrate next month?

Journal your Thoughts of the Month:

_____

_____

_____

Month:

Prompts:

What was good,
What could I have improved on,
What have I enjoyed,
What questions do I need to ask,
Who can I connect with.

Journal your Thoughts of the Month:

_____

_____

_____

_____

_____

_____

_____

_____

_____

_____

_____

_____

_____

_____

_____

_____

My To Do List:

_____
_____
_____
_____
_____
_____
_____
_____
_____
_____
_____
_____

My Personal Affirmation for the month:

Date:

Lets Re Do the Footstep Challenge

Plot by colouring in your level of business and wellbeing in each area on a scale of 1 - 10 (1 being the first foot) considering the following:

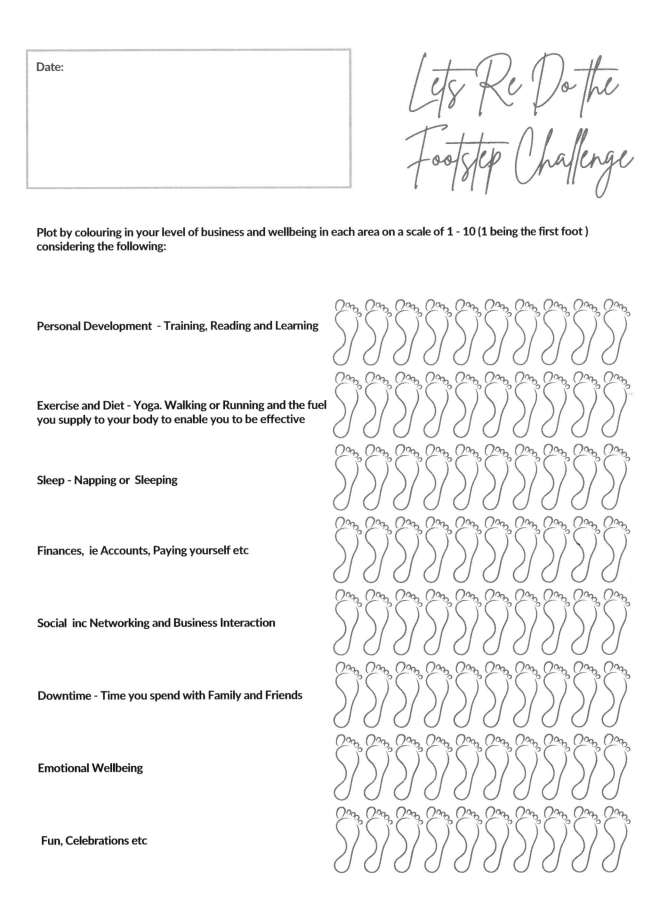

Personal Development - Training, Reading and Learning

Exercise and Diet - Yoga. Walking or Running and the fuel you supply to your body to enable you to be effective

Sleep - Napping or Sleeping

Finances, ie Accounts, Paying yourself etc

Social inc Networking and Business Interaction

Downtime - Time you spend with Family and Friends

Emotional Wellbeing

Fun, Celebrations etc

Month:

Week:

Weekly Business Intentions

I must achieve this week:

1. ....

2. ....

3. ....

4. ....

5. ....

How many followers do you have:

Facebook Page: ....

Facebook Group: ....

Instagram: ....

LinkedIn: ....

Affirmation:

Numbers:

What is my Financial Goal for the week?

How many clients would you like to see?   How many new clients would you like to see?

How will you achieve the numbers above:

....

....

....

Theme for the Week:

Weekly Social Media Planning

What subjects can you break your theme into subjects:

Monday:

Tuesday:

Wednesday:

Thursday:

Friday:

Weekend:

Social Media Locations:

Colour in the hearts when the content is posted or scheduled

	M	T	W	T	F	S	S
Facebook Page	♡	♡	♡	♡	♡	♡	♡
Facebook Group	♡	♡	♡	♡	♡	♡	♡
Facebook Live	♡	♡	♡	♡	♡	♡	♡
Instagram	♡	♡	♡	♡	♡	♡	♡
Instagram Stories	♡	♡	♡	♡	♡	♡	♡
LinkedIn	♡	♡	♡	♡	♡	♡	♡
Twitter	♡	♡	♡	♡	♡	♡	♡
Google	♡	♡	♡	♡	♡	♡	♡

Theme for the week Hashtags:

Month:

Week:

Selfcare Checks:

Colour in the hearts when you have achieved each self care step.

Colour in one for once and both for more than once.

Have you:

Exercised ♡ ♡

Journaled ♡ ♡

Affirmed your Affirmation ♡ ♡

5 minutes Silence ♡ ♡

Visualised where you want to be by the end of the week ♡ ♡

Written down 5 things a day you are grateful for ♡ ♡

Meditation ♡ ♡

Set my Intentions for the week ♡ ♡

Read a book ♡ ♡

I am grateful for:

1.

2.

3.

4.

5.

What will you do to celebrate the week?

What is your ONE selfcare non negotiable this week?

What was your unexpected WIN of the week?

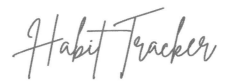

Habit Tracker

Habit trackers are exactly what they say they are. Map out your footsteps to keeping your new habits on track:

Where are you now?

Colour in how well you are doing today

This wheel is the start of your footsteps to creating some great habits to help you keep your business on sturdy footings.

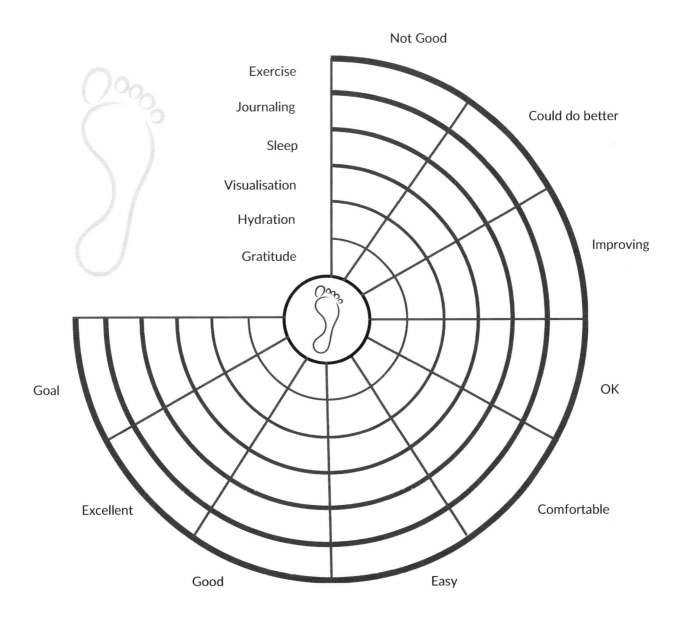

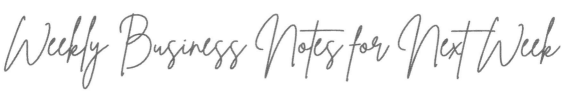

Weekly Business Notes for Next Week

Month:

Week:

Weekly Business Intentions

I must achieve this week:

1. ....

2. ....

3. ....

4. ....

5. ....

How many followers do you have:

Facebook Page: ....

Facebook Group: ....

Instagram: ....

LinkedIn: ....

Affirmation:

Numbers:

What is my Financial Goal for the week?

How many clients would you like to see?   How many new clients would you like to see?

How will you achieve the numbers above:

....

....

....

Theme for the Week:

Weekly Social Media Planning

What subjects can you break your theme into subjects:

Monday:

Tuesday:

Wednesday:

Thursday:

Friday:

Weekend:

Social Media Locations:

Colour in the hearts when the content is posted or scheduled

	M	T	W	T	F	S	S
Facebook Page	♡	♡	♡	♡	♡	♡	♡
Facebook Group	♡	♡	♡	♡	♡	♡	♡
Facebook Live	♡	♡	♡	♡	♡	♡	♡
Instagram	♡	♡	♡	♡	♡	♡	♡
Instagram Stories	♡	♡	♡	♡	♡	♡	♡
LinkedIn	♡	♡	♡	♡	♡	♡	♡
Twitter	♡	♡	♡	♡	♡	♡	♡
Google	♡	♡	♡	♡	♡	♡	♡

Theme for the week Hashtags:

Month:	*Weekly Business*
Week:	*Checks and Selfcare*

Selfcare Checks:

Colour in the hearts when you have achieved each self care step.

Colour in one for once and both for more than once.

Have you:

Exercised ♡ ♡

Journaled ♡ ♡

Affirmed your Affirmation ♡ ♡

5 minutes Silence ♡ ♡

Visualised where you want to be by the end of the week ♡ ♡

Written down 5 things a day you are grateful for ♡ ♡

Meditation ♡ ♡

Set my Intentions for the week ♡ ♡

Read a book ♡ ♡

I am grateful for:

1.

2.

3.

4.

5.

What will you do to celebrate the week?

What is your ONE selfcare non negotiable this week?

What was your unexpected WIN of the week?

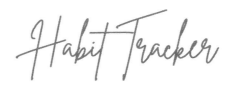

Habit Tracker

Habit trackers are exactly what they say they are. Map out your footsteps to keeping your new habits on track:

Where are you now?

Colour in how well you are doing today

This wheel is the start of your footsteps to creating some great habits to help you keep your business on sturdy footings.

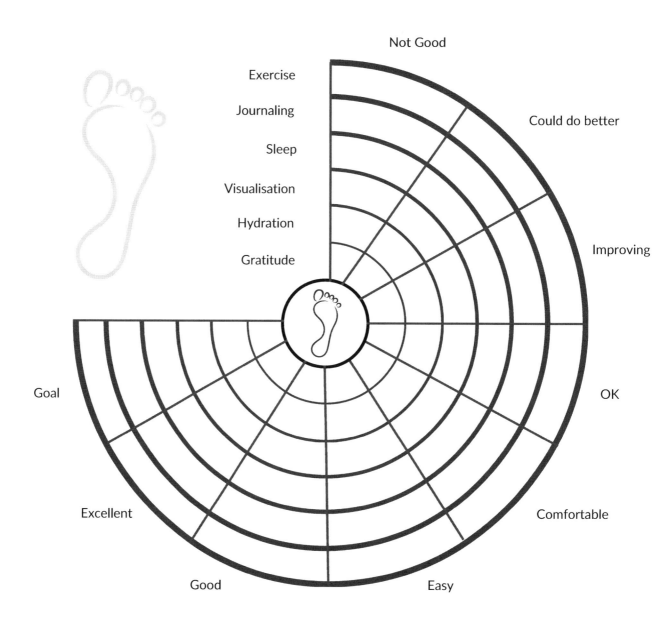

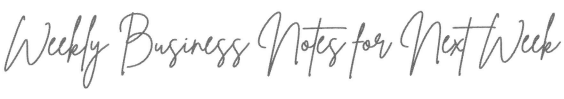

Weekly Business Notes for Next Week

Month:

Week:

Weekly Business Intentions

I must achieve this week:

1. ....

2. ....

3. ....

4. ....

5. ....

How many followers do you have:

Facebook Page: ....

Facebook Group: ....

Instagram: ....

LinkedIn: ....

Affirmation:

Numbers:

What is my Financial Goal for the week?

How many clients would you like to see?   How many new clients would you like to see?

How will you achieve the numbers above:

....

....

....

Theme for the Week:

Weekly Social Media Planning

What subjects can you break your theme into subjects:

Monday:

Tuesday:

Wednesday:

Thursday:

Friday:

Weekend:

Social Media Locations:

Colour in the hearts when the content is posted or scheduled

	M	T	W	T	F	S	S
Facebook Page	♡	♡	♡	♡	♡	♡	♡
Facebook Group	♡	♡	♡	♡	♡	♡	♡
Facebook Live	♡	♡	♡	♡	♡	♡	♡
Instagram	♡	♡	♡	♡	♡	♡	♡
Instagram Stories	♡	♡	♡	♡	♡	♡	♡
LinkedIn	♡	♡	♡	♡	♡	♡	♡
Twitter	♡	♡	♡	♡	♡	♡	♡
Google	♡	♡	♡	♡	♡	♡	♡

Theme for the week Hashtags:

Month:

Week:

Selfcare Checks:

Colour in the hearts when you have achieved each self care step.

Colour in one for once and both for more than once.

Have you:

Exercised ♡ ♡

Journaled ♡ ♡

Affirmed your Affirmation ♡ ♡

5 minutes Silence ♡ ♡

Visualised where you want to be by the end of the week ♡ ♡

Written down 5 things a day you are grateful for ♡ ♡

Meditation ♡ ♡

Set my Intentions for the week ♡ ♡

Read a book ♡ ♡

I am grateful for:

1.

2.

3.

4.

5.

What will you do to celebrate the week?

What is your ONE selfcare non negotiable this week?

What was your unexpected WIN of the week?

Habit Tracker

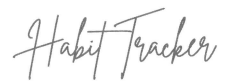

Habit trackers are exactly what they say they are. Map out your footsteps to keeping your new habits on track:

Where are you now?

Colour in how well you are doing today

This wheel is the start of your footsteps to creating some great habits to help you keep your business on sturdy footings.

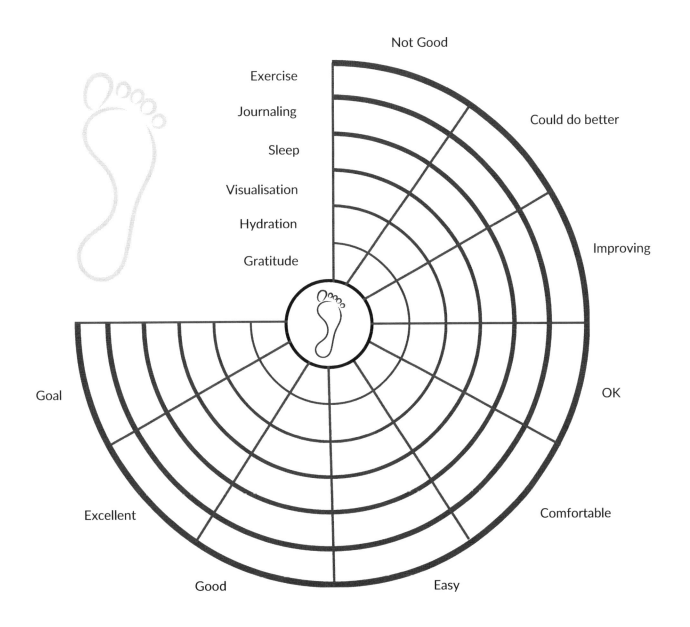

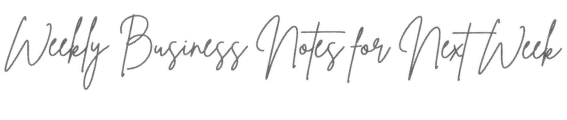

Weekly Business Notes for Next Week

Month:

Week:

Weekly Business Intentions

I must achieve this week:

1. ....

2. ....

3. ....

4. ....

5. ....

How many followers do you have:

Facebook Page: ....

Facebook Group: ....

Instagram: ....

LinkedIn: ....

Affirmation:

Numbers:

What is my Financial Goal for the week?

How many clients would you like to see?   How many new clients would you like to see?

How will you achieve the numbers above:

....

....

....

Theme for the Week:

What subjects can you break your theme into subjects:

Monday:

Tuesday:

Wednesday:

Thursday:

Friday:

Weekend:

Social Media Locations:

Colour in the hearts when the content is posted or scheduled

	M	T	W	T	F	S	S
Facebook Page	♡	♡	♡	♡	♡	♡	♡
Facebook Group	♡	♡	♡	♡	♡	♡	♡
Facebook Live	♡	♡	♡	♡	♡	♡	♡
Instagram	♡	♡	♡	♡	♡	♡	♡
Instagram Stories	♡	♡	♡	♡	♡	♡	♡
LinkedIn	♡	♡	♡	♡	♡	♡	♡
Twitter	♡	♡	♡	♡	♡	♡	♡
Google	♡	♡	♡	♡	♡	♡	♡

Theme for the week Hashtags:

Month:

Week:

Selfcare Checks:

Colour in the hearts when you have achieved each self care step.

Colour in one for once and both for more than once.

Have you:

Exercised ♡ ♡

Journaled ♡ ♡

Affirmed your Affirmation ♡ ♡

5 minutes Silence ♡ ♡

Visualised where you want to be by the end of the week ♡ ♡

Written down 5 things a day you are grateful for ♡ ♡

Meditation ♡ ♡

Set my Intentions for the week ♡ ♡

Read a book ♡ ♡

I am grateful for:

1.

2.

3.

4.

5.

What will you do to celebrate the week?

What is your ONE selfcare non negotiable this week?

What was your unexpected WIN of the week?

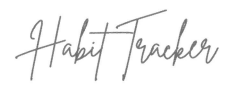

Habit Tracker

Habit trackers are exactly what they say they are. Map out your footsteps to keeping your new habits on track:

Where are you now?

Colour in how well you are doing today

This wheel is the start of your footsteps to creating some great habits to help you keep your business on sturdy footings.

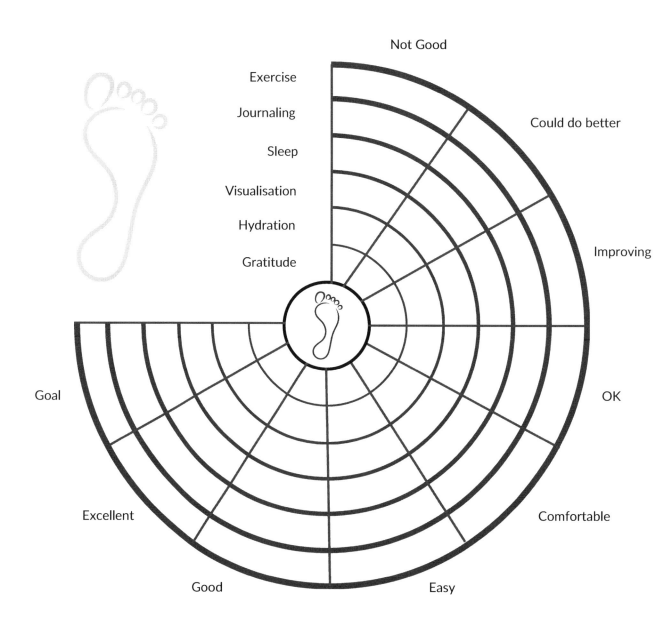

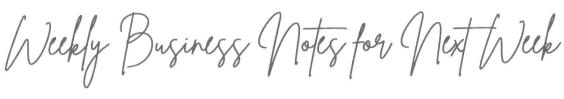

Weekly Business Notes for Next Week

_____

_____

_____

_____

_____

_____

_____

_____

_____

_____

_____

_____

_____

_____

Month:

Week:

Weekly Business Intentions

I must achieve this week:

1. ....

2. ....

3. ....

4. ....

5. ....

How many followers do you have:

Facebook Page: ....

Facebook Group: ....

Instagram: ....

LinkedIn: ....

Affirmation:

Numbers:

What is my Financial Goal for the week?

How many clients would you like to see?   How many new clients would you like to see?

How will you achieve the numbers above:

....

....

....

Theme for the Week:

What subjects can you break your theme into subjects:

Monday:

Tuesday:

Wednesday:

Thursday:

Friday:

Weekend:

Social Media Locations:

Colour in the hearts when the content is posted or scheduled

	M	T	W	T	F	S	S
Facebook Page	♡	♡	♡	♡	♡	♡	♡
Facebook Group	♡	♡	♡	♡	♡	♡	♡
Facebook Live	♡	♡	♡	♡	♡	♡	♡
Instagram	♡	♡	♡	♡	♡	♡	♡
Instagram Stories	♡	♡	♡	♡	♡	♡	♡
LinkedIn	♡	♡	♡	♡	♡	♡	♡
Twitter	♡	♡	♡	♡	♡	♡	♡
Google	♡	♡	♡	♡	♡	♡	♡

Theme for the week Hashtags:

Month:

Week:

Selfcare Checks:

Colour in the hearts when you have achieved each self care step.

Colour in one for once and both for more than once.

Have you:

Exercised ♡ ♡

Journaled ♡ ♡

Affirmed your Affirmation ♡ ♡

5 minutes Silence ♡ ♡

Visualised where you want to be by the end of the week ♡ ♡

Written down 5 things a day you are grateful for ♡ ♡

Meditation ♡ ♡

Set my Intentions for the week ♡ ♡

Read a book ♡ ♡

I am grateful for:

1.

2.

3.

4.

5.

What will you do to celebrate the week?

What is your ONE selfcare non negotiable this week?

What was your unexpected WIN of the week?

Habit Tracker

Habit trackers are exactly what they say they are. Map out your footsteps to keeping your new habits on track:

Where are you now?

Colour in how well you are doing today

This wheel is the start of your footsteps to creating some great habits to help you keep your business on sturdy footings.

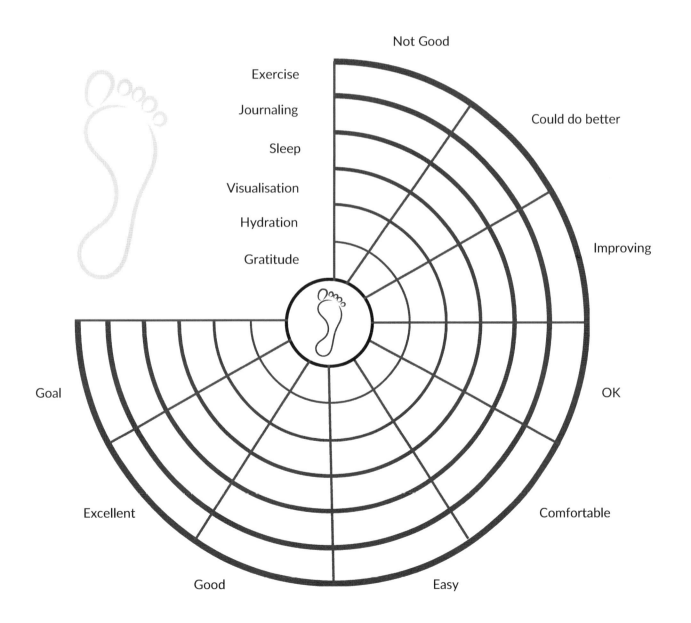

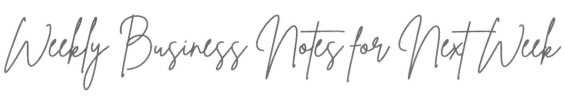

Weekly Business Notes for Next Week

Month:

Week:

Monthly Checks:

Colour in the hearts when you have achieved each self care step.

Have you:

1. Updated your website ♡
2. Written a blog ♡
3. Read an inspirational book ♡
4. Gone "Live" on Facebook ♡
5. Done a "Reel" on Instagram ♡
6. Preschedule your posts for next month ♡
7. Planned your socials for next month ♡
8. Exercised each day/week ♡
9. Increased your Tax Savings Bank Account ♡
10. Booked a month end Celebration ♡
11. Paid all your invoices ♡
12. Are your accounts up to date ♡
13. Did your social media grow ♡
14. Did your client list grow ♡
15. Pay yourself ♡
16. Met up with a business colleague ♡
17. Attended a networking event ♡
18. Organised a treat for YOU ♡
19. Achieved your financial goals ♡
20. Increased your costs per client ♡

This month I am grateful for:

1.

2.

3.

4.

5.

What was your unexpected WIN of the month?

What will you do to celebrate next month?

Journal your Thoughts of the Month:

Month:

Prompts:

What was good,
What could I have improved on,
What have I enjoyed,
What questions do I need to ask,
Who can I connect with.

Journal your Thoughts of the Month:

_____

_____

_____

_____

_____

_____

_____

_____

_____

_____

_____

_____

_____

_____

_____

_____

My To Do List:

_____

_____

_____

_____

_____

_____

_____

_____

_____

_____

_____

_____

My Personal Affirmation for the month:

Date:

Let's Re Do the
Footstep Challenge

Plot by colouring in your level of business and wellbeing in each area on a scale of 1 - 10 (1 being the first foot)
considering the following:

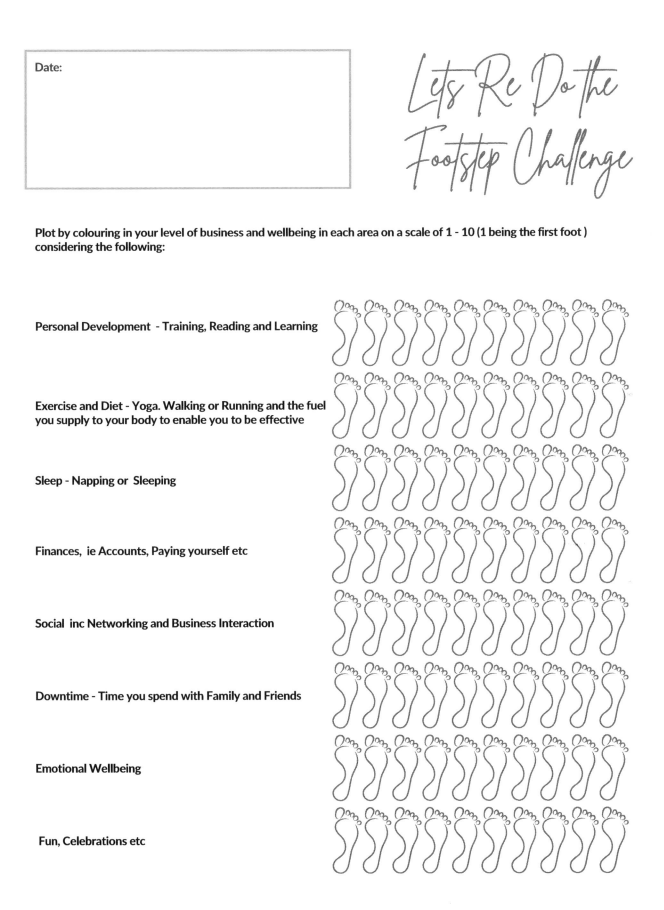

Personal Development - Training, Reading and Learning

Exercise and Diet - Yoga. Walking or Running and the fuel you supply to your body to enable you to be effective

Sleep - Napping or Sleeping

Finances, ie Accounts, Paying yourself etc

Social inc Networking and Business Interaction

Downtime - Time you spend with Family and Friends

Emotional Wellbeing

Fun, Celebrations etc

Quarter :

Months included:

Quarterly Social Media Growth

	Facebook Page A	Facebook Group B	Instagram C	Total A+B+C	Growth on previous month
Week 1					0
Week 2					
Week 3					
Week 4					
Week 5					
Week 6					
Week 7					
Week 8					
Week 9					
Week 10					
Week 11					
Week 12					
TOTALS					

Quarter :

Months included:

Quarterly Clients & Turnover Growth

	No of Clients A	No of New Clients B	WeeklyTurnover C	Turnover per client C/A
Week 1				
Week 2				
Week 3				
Week 4				
Week 5				
Week 6				
Week 7				
Week 8				
Week 9				
Week 10				
Week 11				
Week 12				
TOTALS				

Journal your Thoughts of the Quarter:

_____

_____

_____

_____

Month:

Prompts in 3 moths time:

Where do you want to be
What do you want to have achieved
What do you want to learn
Do you need to research a course

_____

_____

_____

_____

_____

_____

_____

_____

_____

_____

_____

_____

_____

_____

_____

Journal your Thoughts of the Quarter:

_____

_____

_____

_____

_____

_____

_____

_____

_____

_____

_____

_____

_____

_____

_____

_____

_____

My To Do List

BUSINESS:

_____
_____
_____
_____
_____
_____
_____
_____
_____
_____
_____
_____
_____
_____

PERSONAL:

_____
_____
_____
_____
_____
_____
_____
_____
_____

Well Done

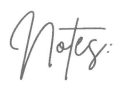

Notes:

Notes:

My To Do List

LEARNING:

_____
_____
_____
_____
_____
_____
_____
_____
_____
_____
_____
_____
_____

VISIBILITY:

_____
_____
_____
_____
_____
_____
_____
_____
_____

Well Done

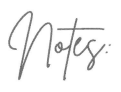

Notes:

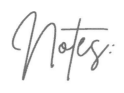

Notes:

My To Do List

LEARNING:

VISIBILITY:

Well Done

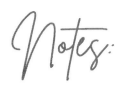

Notes:

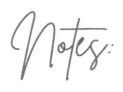

Notes:

My To Do List

LEARNING:

VISIBILITY:

well done

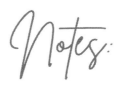

Notes:

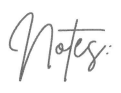

Notes:

My To Do List

LEARNING:

VISIBILITY:

Well Done

My To Do List

LEARNING:

VISIBILITY:

Well Done

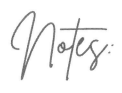

Notes:

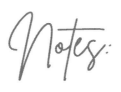
Notes:

My To Do List

LEARNING:

VISIBILITY:

Well Done

Gratitude

 First, thank you for using The Reflexology Planner, I hope that you have found it useful and eye opening. Maybe you will be purchasing another one to complete the year.

 Secondly, thank you, for working with the planner from start to finish. I hope you have seen just how awesome you are. Your journey is only just beginning.

 Finally, if you would like to work with me on a 121 basis or as part of a small group. Please get in touch via Facebook @findingmyfeet or email katie@katiepage.co.uk

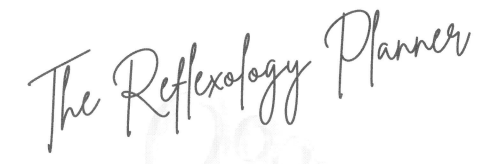

The Reflexology Planner

I do hope that you have enjoyed and found using
The Reflexology Planner useful.

I have carefully chosen the subjects and the titles to go inside as
being the most relevant to a Reflexologist wishing to nurture and
grow their reflexology business.

As I practice Gratitude throughout my planner, I wish to say
THANK YOU. Thank you for taking the time out to buy "The
Reflexology Planner", using it and feeding back your thoughts.

If you have liked working with the planner and wish to work with
me more please check out my website.

www.katiepage.co.uk

Facebook: @katiepagereflexology
Facebook Group: @findingmyfeet

Instagram: @katiepagereflexology

Printed in Great Britain
by Amazon

65087614R00127